CASE REVIEW
Cardiac Imaging
Second Edition

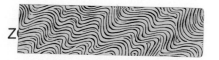

Series Editor
David M. Yousem, MD, MBA
Professor of Radiology
Director of Neuroradiology
Russell H. Morgan Department of Radiology and Radiological Science
The Johns Hopkins Medical Institutions
Baltimore, Maryland

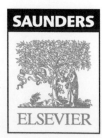

SAUNDERS

ELSEVIER

Gautham P. Reddy, MD, MPH
Professor of Radiology
Vice Chair for Education
Director of Thoracic Imaging
University of Washington
Seattle, Washington

Robert M. Steiner, MD, FACC
Professor of Radiology
Director, Thoracic Radiology
Temple University Hospital
Philadelphia, Pennsylvania

Christopher M. Walker, MD
Assistant Professor
Department of Radiology
University of Missouri-Kansas City School of Medicine
Cardiothoracic Radiologist
Saint Luke's Hospital of Kansas City
Kansas City, Missouri

CASE REVIEW

Cardiac Imaging

SECOND EDITION

CASE REVIEW SERIES

1600 John F. Kennedy Blvd.
Ste 1800
Philadelphia, PA 19103-2899

CARDIAC IMAGING: CASE REVIEW SERIES, SECOND EDITION   ISBN: 978-0-323-06519-1

Notice

Knowledge and best practice in this field are constantly changing. As new research and experience broaden our understanding, changes in research methods, professional practices, or medical treatment may become necessary.

Practitioners and researchers must always rely on their own experience and knowledge in evaluating and using any information, methods, compounds, or experiments described herein. In using such information or methods they should be mindful of their own safety and the safety of others, including parties for whom they have a professional responsibility.

With respect to any drug or pharmaceutical products identified, readers are advised to check the most current information provided (i) on procedures featured or (ii) by the manufacturer of each product to be administered, to verify the recommended dose or formula, the method and duration of administration, and contraindications. It is the responsibility of practitioners, relying on their own experience and knowledge of their patients, to make diagnoses, to determine dosages and the best treatment for each individual patient, and to take all appropriate safety precautions.

To the fullest extent of the law, neither the Publisher nor the authors, contributors, or editors assume any liability for any injury and/or damage to persons or property as a matter of products liability, negligence or otherwise, or from any use or operation of any methods, products, instructions, or ideas contained in the material herein.

Library of Congress Cataloging-in-Publication Data
Reddy, Gautham P., author.
  Cardiac imaging : case review / Gautham P. Reddy, Robert M. Steiner, Christopher M. Walker.
- Second edition.
    p. ; cm. – (Case review series)
  Includes bibliographical references and index.
  ISBN 978-0-323-06519-1 (pbk. : alk. paper)
  I. Steiner, Robert M., author. II. Walker, Christopher M., author. III. Title. IV. Series: Case review series.
  [DNLM: 1. Cardiac Imaging Techniques–methods–Problems and Exercises. 2. Cardiovascular Diseases–radiography–Problems and Exercises. WG 18.2]
  RC683.5.R3
  616.1´207540076-dc23

                                                      2013033292

Senior Content Strategist: Don Scholz
Content Development Specialist: Katy Meert
Publishing Services Manager: Deborah L. Vogel
Project Manager: Bridget Healy
Design Direction: Steven Stave

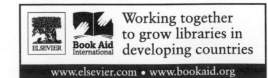

To Gayatri, Maurya, and Kaniska
GPR

To Marilyn, Emily, Peter, and Sophia
RMS

To Eunhee, a fantastic mother and my best friend.
To Elsie and Lillian, the best daughters a father could ask for.
CMW

I have been very gratified by the popularity and positive feedback that the authors of the Case Review Series have received on the publication of the editions of their volumes. Reviews in journals and online sites as well as word-of-mouth comments have been uniformly favorable. The authors have done an outstanding job in filling the niche of an affordable, easy-to-access, case-based learning tool that supplements the material in The Requisites series. I have been told by residents, fellows, and practicing radiologists that the Case Review Series books are the ideal means for studying for oral board examinations and subspecialty certification tests.

Although some students learn best in a non-interactive study book mode, others need the anxiety or excitement of being quizzed. The selected format for the Case Review series (which consists of showing a few images needed to construct a differential diagnosis and then asking a few clinical and imaging questions) was designed to simulate the board examination experience. The only difference is that the Case Review books provide the correct answer and immediate feedback. The limit and range of the reader's knowledge are tested through scaled cases ranging from relatively easy to very hard. The Case Review Series also offers a brief discussion of each case, a link back to the pertinent The Requisites volume, and up-to-date references from the literature.

Because of the popularity of online learning, we have been rolling out new editions on the web. We also have adjusted to the new Boards format which will be electronic and largely case-based. We are ready for the new boards! The Case Review questions have been reframed into multiple-choice format, the links are dynamic to online references, and feedback is interactive with correct and incorrect answers. Personally, I am very excited about the future. Join us.

David M. Yousem, MD, MBA

Cardiac Imaging, 2ⁿᵈ edition by Drs. Reddy, Steiner, and Walker explores advanced cardiac imaging including coronary and pulmonary artery CT angiography, cardiac MRI, and nuclear medicine applications. These studies are increasingly being performed emergently in the Emergency Department as part of the chest pain work up. Radiologists have been able, thru excellent training and technique advancement, to maintain a strong influence in this arena and share the spotlight with cardiologists. It is essential that we radiologists learn the anatomy and pathology as well as our clinical colleagues.

The authors have compiled a wonderful array of cases that demonstrate the power of various modalities in our imaging armamentarium. There is an emphasis on differential diagnosis, multiple choice questions, and a summary of relevant information on the entity. I expect that this edition will be the "study of choice" for residents preparing for the new boards format.

I congratulate Drs. Reddy, Steiner, and Walker for maintaining the outstanding quality of the Case Review Series and modernizing it for the online learning environment.

David M. Yousem, MD, MBA
Case Review Series Editor

Since the first edition of *Cardiac Imaging* was published in 2006, the interest in cardiovascular imaging by practicing radiologists, residents-in-training, and cardiologists has greatly increased. Indications for advanced cardiac imaging utilizing MRI, CT, PET, and Echocardiography have broadened considerably, and imaging techniques have significantly improved. With the changes in the board examinations in radiology; expanding interest in certification in cardiovascular imaging by practicing physicians; and the increasing demands for expertise in cardiac imaging among radiology groups, expansion of the case selection in this second edition is particularly relevant.

In this revision, we included most of the topics and related images from the first edition and added a number of new examples of both common conditions and the more unusual disease entities that will be found in a busy clinical practice (and in the imaging board and other qualifying examinations).

The case selection now includes a greater number of multimodality examples of congenital cardiovascular disease, ischemic and non-ischemic cardiomyopathies, and vascular conditions including coronary, aortic, and pulmonary vascular disease. Advanced imaging techniques such as velocity-encoded cine MRI, and delayed enhancement strategies with CT and MRI are included.

As in the first edition, the case book is divided into three sections: Opening Round, Fair Game, and Challenge cases. Opening Round cases are straightforward and shouldn't be too difficult for most trainees and experienced imagers. Fair Game cases will generally require a greater knowledge base. Challenge cases will be more complex, of rarer incidence, and may require advanced imaging techniques.

We are confident that you will find this second edition of *Cardiac Imaging* to be a valuable addition to your library and add to your knowledge of cardiovascular imaging.

Gautham P. Reddy
Robert M. Steiner
Christopher M. Walker

Opening Round

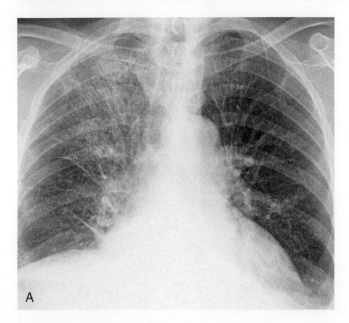

A

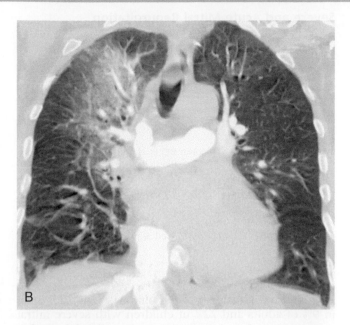

B

History: No patient history is available.

1. What should be included in the differential diagnosis for ground-glass opacity? (Choose all that apply.)
   A. Pulmonary edema
   B. Pneumonia
   C. Pulmonary hemorrhage
   D. Adenocarcinoma in situ (bronchioloalveolar cell carcinoma)

2. If this patient presented with fever and a productive cough, what is the most likely diagnosis?
   A. Right upper lobe pulmonary edema
   B. Atypical pneumonia
   C. Pulmonary hemorrhage
   D. Adenocarcinoma in situ (bronchioloalveolar cell carcinoma)

3. If this patient presented with severe chest pain and no infectious symptoms, what would be the most likely diagnosis?
   A. Right upper lobe pulmonary edema
   B. Atypical pneumonia
   C. Pulmonary hemorrhage
   D. Adenocarcinoma in situ (bronchioloalveolar cell carcinoma)

4. If acute mitral regurgitation is the suspected diagnosis based on the chest radiograph and clinical presentation, what is the next best step in management?
   A. CT
   B. Echocardiography
   C. Follow-up radiograph
   D. MRI

Severe and Acute Mitral Regurgitation

1. A, B, C, and D

2. B

3. A

4. B

Reference

Schnyder PA, Sarraj AM, Duvoisin BE, et al: Pulmonary edema associated with mitral regurgitation: prevalence of predominant involvement of the right upper lobe, *AJR Am J Roentgenol* 161(1):33–36, 1993.

Cross-Reference

Cardiac Imaging: The REQUISITES, ed 3, pp 191-194.

Comment

Pathophysiology

Asymmetric right upper lobe pulmonary edema is seen in 9% of adults and 22% of children with severe mitral regurgitation. In adults, it is usually caused by a flail posterior valve leaflet secondary to myocardial infarction. A flail posterior leaflet causes the mitral regurgitant jet to be preferentially directed into the right superior pulmonary vein; this leads to focal increased hydrostatic pressure and pulmonary edema within the right upper lobe. In the setting of chest pain, acute mitral regurgitation must be considered and can be confirmed with echocardiography.

Imaging

The radiograph (Fig. A) and CT scan (Fig. B) show asymmetric right upper lobe ground-glass opacity. The differential diagnosis varies depending on the patient's clinical presentation. In the setting of fever and productive cough, the imaging findings are consistent with atypical pneumonia. In this case, the patient had severe chest pain and acute myocardial infarction. Echocardiography confirmed severe mitral regurgitation.

Notes

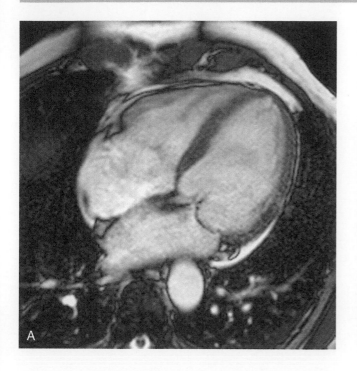

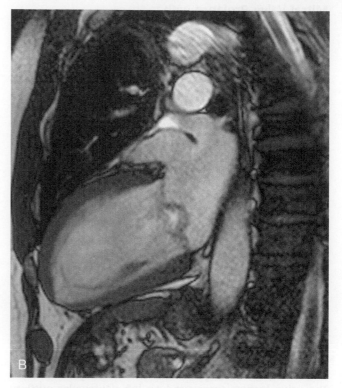

History: A patient presents with cardiac arrhythmia and undergoes evaluation for arrhythmogenic right ventricular dysplasia.

1. What should be included in the differential diagnosis for mitral regurgitation? (Choose all that apply.)
   A. Mitral valve prolapse
   B. Myocardial ischemia
   C. Dilated cardiomyopathy
   D. Endocarditis

2. What is the most likely diagnosis?
   A. Mitral valve prolapse
   B. Myocardial ischemia
   C. Dilated cardiomyopathy
   D. Endocarditis

3. Which imaging plane is ideal for diagnosing this condition?
   A. Four-chamber
   B. Short-axis
   C. Left ventricular outflow tract (3-chamber)
   D. Right ventricular outflow tract

4. Which of the following is a potential complication of this condition?
   A. Aortic dissection
   B. Mitral stenosis
   C. Arrhythmia
   D. Patent foramen ovale

Mitral Valve Prolapse with Mitral Regurgitation

1. A, B, C, and D

2. A

3. C

4. C

References

Feuchtner GM, Alkadhi H, Karlo C, et al: Cardiac CT angiography for the diagnosis of mitral valve prolapse: comparison with echocardiography, *Radiology* 254(2):374-383, 2010.

Han Y, Peters DC, Salton CJ, et al: Cardiovascular magnetic resonance characterization of mitral valve prolapse, *JACC Cardiovasc Imaging* 1(3):294-303, 2008.

Cross-Reference

Cardiac Imaging: The REQUISITES, ed 3, pp 192-193.

Comment

Epidemiology

Mitral valve prolapse affects 2% to 3% of the population and is the most common cause of severe nonischemic mitral regurgitation requiring surgery (Fig. A). It is defined by greater than 2 mm of atrial displacement of the valve leaflets (measured on left ventricular outflow tract or vertical long-axis [2-chamber] images) with respect to the mitral anulus (Fig. B). There are two types of mitral valve prolapse: billowing (as shown in this case) and flail leaflet (caused by chordal rupture secondary to endocarditis or rheumatic heart disease). Mitral valve prolapse is most commonly due to myxomatous degeneration of mitral leaflets but can also be seen in patients with atrial secundum septal defects, connective tissue disorders, and recent diuretic use.

Imaging

Mitral valve prolapse may be incorrectly diagnosed if only four-chamber images are viewed secondary to the natural saddle shape of the mitral anulus. Myxomatous leaflet (defined as a leaflet thickness measuring >5 mm) predisposes patients to fatal arrhythmia, severe mitral regurgitation, and endocarditis. It is important to identify mitral valve prolapse on cardiac CT or MRI examinations performed for other reasons because these patients may benefit from endocarditis prophylaxis or anticoagulation therapy.

Notes

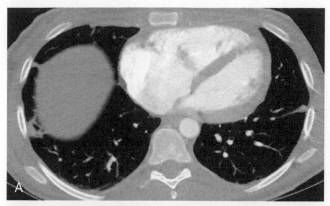

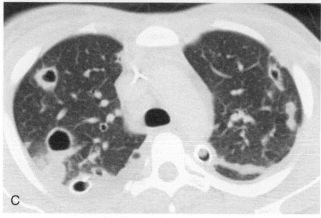

History: A patient presents with chest pain.

1. What should be included in the differential
   diagnosis of a valvular mass? (Choose all that apply.)
   A. Angiosarcoma
   B. Thrombus
   C. Vegetation
   D. Myxoma
   E. Papillary fibroelastoma

2. What is the most common valvular tumor?
   A. Thrombus
   B. Papillary fibroelastoma
   C. Myxoma
   D. Angiosarcoma

3. What is the most likely diagnosis?
   A. Wegener granulomatosis
   B. Angioinvasive aspergillosis
   C. Septic pulmonary embolism
   D. Papillary fibroelastoma

4. In regard to this diagnosis, which valve is most
   commonly affected in intravenous drug users?
   A. Aortic valve
   B. Mitral valve
   C. Pulmonary valve
   D. Tricuspid valve

Septic Pulmonary Embolism with Tricuspid Valve Endocarditis

1. A, B, C, D, and E

2. B

3. C

4. D

Reference

Feuchtner GM, Stolzmann P, Dichtl W, et al: Multislice computed tomography in infective endocarditis: comparison with transesophageal echocardiography and intraoperative findings, *J Am Coll Cardiol* 53(5):436-444, 2009.

Cross-Reference

Cardiac Imaging: The REQUISITES, ed 3, p 283.

Comment

Imaging

Prospectively gated cardiac CT scan through the level of the tricuspid valve shows an oval-shaped mass (Figs. A and B). CT scan at a higher level with lung windows (Fig. C) shows multiple peripherally located cavitary lung nodules. This patient was an intravenous drug user who presented with high fever and sepsis. Findings are consistent with septic pulmonary embolism from a tricuspid valve vegetation.

Differential Diagnosis

The differential diagnosis for a valvular mass is limited. In the setting of intravenous drug use, the most common valvular mass is a vegetation. Gated CT is both sensitive and specific for detecting a valvular vegetation in patients with suspected endocarditis. CT may be better suited than transesophageal or transthoracic echocardiography to help with surgical planning because it better delineates the anatomic structures involved by a potential perivalvular abscess or pseudoaneurysm. In the absence of infectious symptoms, a valvular mass is most likely tumor or thrombus. The most common valvular tumor is papillary fibroelastoma. This tumor may be seen only on echocardiography because it is usually small (<1 cm) and very mobile. A valvular tumor is best differentiated from valvular thrombus because a tumor demonstrates contrast enhancement on either CT or MRI.

Notes

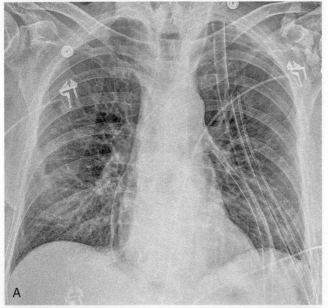

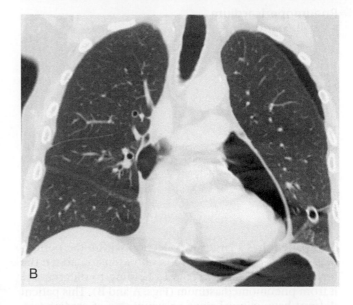

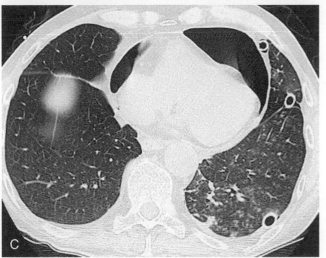

History: A patient presents with chest pain.

1. What should be included in the differential
   diagnosis for air adjacent to the heart seen on the
   chest radiograph? (Choose all that apply.)
   A. Pneumopericardium
   B. Pneumothorax
   C. Pneumoperitoneum
   D. Pneumomediastinum

2. What is the most common cause of this entity?
   A. Trauma or iatrogenic
   B. Tumor
   C. Infection
   D. Pneumoperitoneum

3. What would be the best next step in management if
   this patient were hypotensive and bradycardic?
   A. High-flow oxygen (10 L/min)
   B. Serial chest radiographs
   C. Echocardiography
   D. Emergent pericardiocentesis

4. What is the likely mechanism by which barotrauma
   causes this condition?
   A. Pneumothorax
   B. Air dissects along the pulmonary vessels
   C. Low pressure
   D. Puncture of the trachea

Pneumopericardium

1. A, B, and D

2. A

3. D

4. B

Reference

Katabathina VS, Restrepo CS, Martinez-Jimenez S, et al: Nonvascular, nontraumatic mediastinal emergencies in adults: a comprehensive review of imaging findings, *Radiographics* 31(4):1141–1160, 2011.

Comment

Imaging

This patient has a large air collection within the pericardial space (Figs. A-C). There is no extension above the level of the pericardial recesses helping to differentiate it from pneumomediastinum (Figs. A and B). This patient did not have clinical signs or symptoms of cardiac tamponade, and serial imaging (not shown) showed resolution of air.

Diagnosis

Pneumopericardium is most commonly caused by trauma. Nontraumatic causes include infective pericarditis with a gas-forming organism, fistulous communication with the gastrointestinal tract or lung, and extension of pneumomediastinum into the pericardial space. Tension pneumopericardium is a life-threatening condition diagnosed in the setting of hemodynamic collapse. Imaging findings on CT or MRI that suggest tamponade physiology include compression of the anterior aspect of the heart, dilated inferior vena cava, and compression or displacement of cardiac chambers. Immediate pericardial decompression is required in patients with cardiac tamponade to prevent death.

Notes

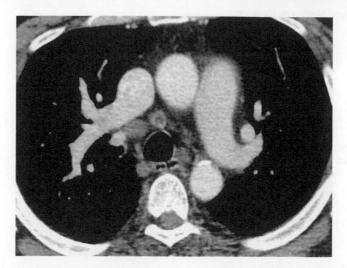

History: A 58-year-old man presents with progressive dyspnea on exertion.

1. What should be included in the differential diagnosis for a left-to-right shunt? (Choose all that apply.)
   A. Partial anomalous pulmonary venous return (PAPVR)
   B. Tetralogy of Fallot
   C. Atrial septal defect (ASD)
   D. Eisenmenger syndrome

2. What is the cardiac abnormality most commonly associated with this condition?
   A. Sinus venosus ASD
   B. Septum primum ASD
   C. Septum secundum ASD
   D. Unroofed coronary sinus

3. Which syndrome or complex is always associated with this entity?
   A. Hypoplastic left heart
   B. Holt-Oram
   C. Scimitar
   D. Carney

4. At which pulmonic-to-systemic flow (Qp/Qs) ratio is repair generally recommended?
   A. 1
   B. 0.3
   C. 1.7
   D. The Qp/Qs ratio is not used to decide when to repair this lesion

Partial Anomalous Pulmonary Venous Return

1. A and C

2. A

3. C

4. C

Reference

Ho ML, Bhalla S, Bierhals A, et al: MDCT of partial anomalous pulmonary venous return (PAPVR) in adults, *J Thorac Imaging* 24(2): 89-95, 2009.

Cross-Reference

Cardiac Imaging: The REQUISITES, ed 3, pp 330-335.

Comment

Epidemiology and Treatment

PAPVR is an uncommon congenital venous anomaly, which occurs in less than 1% of the population. It is a left-to-right shunt with a pulmonary vein or veins bypassing the systemic circulation. When discovered in children, it overwhelmingly affects the right upper lobe (90% of cases) and is highly associated with other cardiac malformations including sinus venosus ASD. Repair of PAPVR is recommended when the Qp/Qs ratio exceeds 1.5 to 2.0. Most children meet these criteria, and usually both ASD and PAPVR are surgically corrected.

Adult Presentation and Management

PAPVR is discovered in adults incidentally on imaging performed for other reasons. It is frequently asymptomatic and most commonly affects the left upper lobe (47%) followed by the right upper lobe (38%). Sinus venosus ASD occurs in 42% of cases of adult right upper lobe PAPVR. Surgery is often not needed in adults because they are asymptomatic.

Imaging

Axial CT shows a right superior pulmonary vein draining directly into the superior vena cava (Figure), consistent with PAPVR. Images more inferior at the level of the upper left atrium (not shown) did not reveal a sinus venosus ASD in this case.

Notes

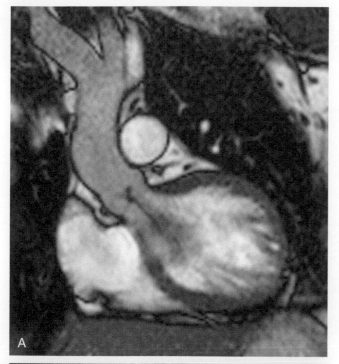

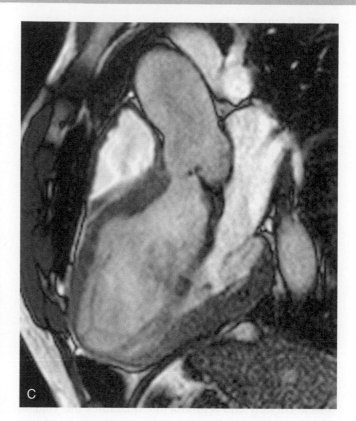

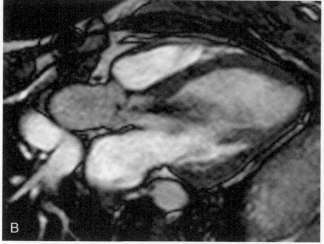

History: Two patients present with progressive dyspnea on exertion.

1. What should be included in the differential diagnosis for these two patients? (Choose all that apply.)
   A. Aortic dissection
   B. Marfan syndrome
   C. Hypertrophic cardiomyopathy
   D. Tetralogy of Fallot repair
   E. Rheumatic heart disease

2. What physical fluid property is responsible for the signal void (black signal) that is seen directed into the left ventricle from the aortic valve?
   A. Steady flow
   B. Laminar flow
   C. Stationary flow
   D. Turbulent flow

3. What is the most frequent cause of the finding in Figs. A-C?
   A. Annuloaortic ectasia
   B. Idiopathic valvular degeneration
   C. Aortic dissection
   D. Endocarditis

4. Which imaging sequence could quantify the abnormality shown in Figs. A-C?
   A. First-pass imaging
   B. Delayed contrast imaging
   C. Black blood T1-weighted imaging
   D. Velocity-encoded cine phase contrast imaging

Aortic Regurgitation

1. A, B, and E

2. D

3. B

4. D

Reference

Glockner JF, Johnston DL, McGee KP: Evaluation of cardiac valvular disease with MR imaging: qualitative and quantitative techniques, *Radiographics* 23(1):e9, 2003.

Cross-Reference

Cardiac Imaging: The REQUISITES, ed 3, pp 182–185.

Comment

Epidemiology

Aortic regurgitation most commonly occurs in elderly patients with senile degeneration of the aortic valve and is often seen in association with aortic stenosis. In patients younger than 40 years of age, aortic regurgitation is often due to Marfan syndrome with aortic root dilation. MRI is ideally suited not only to quantify the volume of regurgitation but also to determine its overall effect on the heart. Velocity-encoded cine phase contrast MRI accurately and reproducibly quantifies the volume of valve regurgitation through measurement of the regurgitant fraction (regurgitant volume/forward stroke volume). Cine SSFP images are able to evaluate the overall effect of the regurgitant valve on the heart through measurement of chamber size, ejection fraction, and cardiac mass. Some authors advocate valve replacement in asymptomatic patients because irreversible damage and ventricular remodeling may have already occurred if the valve is replaced after onset of symptoms.

Imaging

Coronal aorta and left ventricular outflow tract (3-chamber) cine SSFP images (Figs. A-C) show a signal void jet originating from the aortic valve directed posteriorly into the left ventricle. This imaging appearance is consistent with aortic regurgitation.

Notes

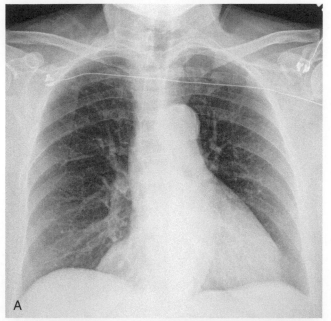

A

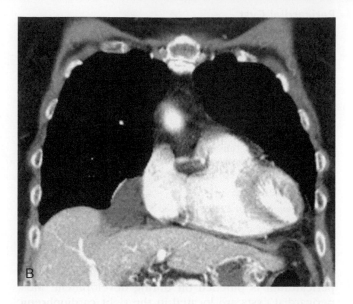

B

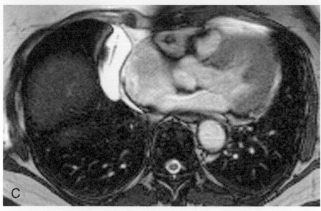

C

History: A patient undergoes preoperative chest radiography before cardiac surgery.

1. What should be included in the differential diagnosis for Fig. A? (Choose all that apply.)
   A. Fat pad
   B. Bronchogenic cyst
   C. Pericardial cyst
   D. Esophageal duplication cyst
   E. Bochdalek hernia

2. Where does this lesion most commonly occur?
   A. Right cardiophrenic angle
   B. Subcarinal space
   C. Anterior mediastinum
   D. Retrocardiac space

3. What is the most likely internal composition of this lesion?
   A. Fat
   B. Soft tissue
   C. Fluid
   D. Calcium

4. What is the next step in management in this asymptomatic patient?
   A. Nothing
   B. Aspiration
   C. Surgical resection
   D. Radiographic follow-up

Pericardial Cyst

1. A and C

2. A

3. C

4. A

Reference

Wang ZJ, Reddy GP, Gotway MB, et al: CT and MR imaging of pericardial disease, *Radiographics* 23 Spec No:S167–S180, 2003.

Cross-Reference

Cardiac Imaging: The REQUISITES, ed 3, pp 56, 78–80, 139–141, 277.

Comment

Epidemiology

Pericardial cysts are congenital lesions formed when pericardium is pinched off during development. Most pericardial cysts are located in the right cardiophrenic angle followed by the left cardiophrenic angle. Cysts can be readily distinguished from other cardiophrenic angle masses with cross-sectional imaging (either CT or MRI). Pericardial cysts are well-defined, nonenhancing lesions of fluid attenuation. They are uniformly hyperintense on T2-weighted MRI.

Presentation

Patients with pericardial cysts are usually asymptomatic, but large cysts can cause dyspnea, chest pain, cough, and rarely cardiac tamponade. Treatment of symptomatic lesions is surgical resection or percutaneous drainage.

Imaging

The chest radiograph shows a well-defined right cardiophrenic angle mass (Fig. A). Coronal CT scan (Fig. B) shows a mass with fluid attenuation and no perceptible wall. Axial T2-weighted MRI (Fig. C) confirms uniform high signal within the lesion.

Notes

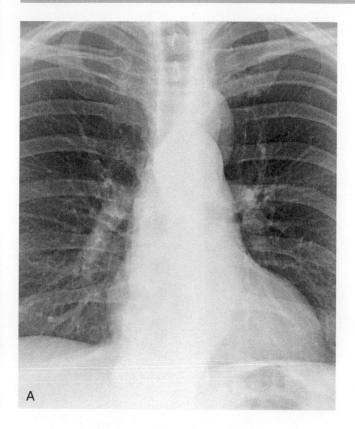

A

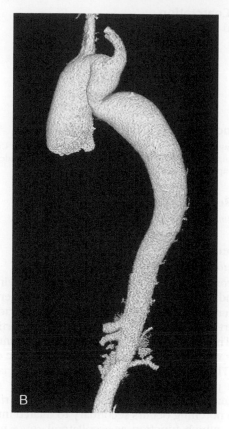

B

History: No patient history is available.

1. What should be included in the differential diagnosis? (Choose all that apply.)
   A. Aortic pseudoaneurysm
   B. Pseudocoarctation
   C. Descending thoracic aortic aneurysm
   D. Aortic coarctation
   E. Traumatic aortic injury

2. Which of the following conditions is most commonly associated with this lesion?
   A. Turner syndrome
   B. Intracranial aneurysm
   C. Bacterial endocarditis
   D. Bicuspid aortic valve

3. What sign or symptom is this patient most likely to have?
   A. Hypertension
   B. Chest pain
   C. Transient ischemic attack
   D. Midsystolic click

4. Which modality provides the most helpful information in diagnosing this condition?
   A. Chest radiograph
   B. MRI
   C. CT
   D. Scintigraphy

CASE 8

Aortic Coarctation

1. B and D

2. D

3. A

4. B

Reference

Kimura-Hayama ET, Meléndez G, Mendizábal AL, et al: Uncommon congenital and acquired aortic diseases: role of multidetector CT angiography, *Radiographics* 30(1):79–98, 2010.

Cross-Reference

Cardiac Imaging: The REQUISITES, ed 3, pp 419–424.

Comment

Epidemiology

Aortic coarctation represents a discrete narrowing of the aorta and is usually juxtaductal in location when discovered later in life. Multiple signs on the chest radiograph may alert the radiologist to the presence of aortic coarctation. The "figure 3" sign represents an abnormal aortic contour with a sharp point occurring at the site of coarctation. This sign occurs in 60% of cases and is usually seen in patients with adult-type coarctation. An additional imaging sign is the presence of inferior rib notching. Rib notching occurs secondary to dilated intercostal arteries, which function as a collateral route for blood flow around the site of aortic narrowing. The main pathway of collateral flow proceeds as follows: aortic arch to subclavian artery to internal mammary artery to intercostal artery to descending thoracic aorta. Additional collateral pathways around the coarctation include the thyrocervical, thoracoacromial trunk, and epigastric arteries.

Associations

The most common association with coarctation is a bicuspid aortic valve followed by Turner syndrome. Aortic coarctation is frequently fatal if it is left untreated. Causes of death include congestive heart failure, aortic dissection, endocarditis, and aortic rupture. Patients are also predisposed to cerebral aneurysms with intracranial hemorrhage owing to carotid artery hypertension.

Imaging

Chest radiography shows a mildly enlarged distal aortic arch that abruptly comes to a sharp point consistent with the "figure 3" sign of aortic coarctation (Fig. A). Volume-rendered CT angiography (Fig. B) also shows the typical "figure 3" sign. The narrowing is distal to the left subclavian artery.

Differential Diagnosis

The main differential diagnosis is aortic pseudocoarctation. MRI is helpful in distinguishing between these two conditions because pseudocoarctation is not associated with a pressure gradient or collateral flow around the narrowed segment.

Notes

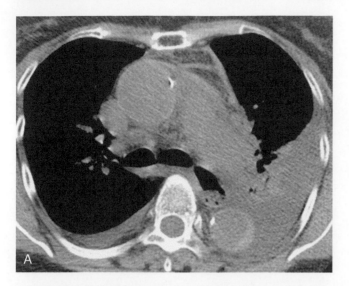

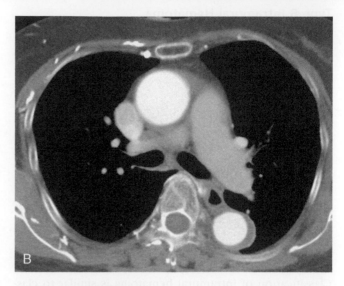

History: The patient presents with tearing chest pain.

1. What should be included in the differential diagnosis of the acute aortic syndrome? (Choose all that apply.)
   A. Aortic dissection
   B. Severe aortic regurgitation
   C. Intramural hematoma
   D. Unstable angina
   E. Penetrating aortic ulcer

2. What is the finding?
   A. Aortic dissection
   B. Descending thoracic aortic aneurysm
   C. Penetrating aortic ulcer
   D. Intramural hematoma

3. How should this abnormality be classified?
   A. Stanford type B
   B. Stanford type A
   C. DeBakey type I
   D. DeBakey type II

4. What is the appropriate management of this patient?
   A. Surgery
   B. Nothing
   C. Medical and conservative management
   D. Endovascular therapy

CASE 9

Type B Intramural Hematoma

1. A, C, and E

2. D

3. A

4. C

Reference

Baikoussis NG, Apostolakis EE, Siminelakis SN, et al: Intramural haematoma of the thoracic aorta: who's to be alerted the cardiologist or the cardiac surgeon? *J Cardiothorac Surg* 4:54, 2009.

Cross-Reference

Cardiac Imaging: The REQUISITES, ed 3, pp 407–411.

Comment

Classification and Management

Classification of intramural hematoma is similar to classification of aortic dissection; intramural hematoma involving the ascending aorta is Stanford type A, and intramural hematoma not involving the ascending aorta is Stanford type B. Differentiation between these two types is important because it determines the most appropriate treatment and is predictive of prognosis. Type A intramural hematoma has a high rate of complications (aortic rupture, pericardial tamponade, progression to aortic dissection, and death) and is generally treated surgically. Type B hematomas infrequently have complications, often resolve without intervention, and are usually managed conservatively. Occasionally, complicated type B intramural hematoma may require surgical or endograft therapy.

Complications

Intramural hematoma is caused by rupture of the vasa vasorum leading to bleeding within the media of the aortic wall. In contrast to aortic dissection, there is no intimal tear. The main complications of intramural hematoma include aortic rupture, hemorrhagic pericardial tamponade, progression to aortic dissection, and aneurysm formation.

Imaging

In this case, non–contrast-enhanced CT scan showed a crescent of high density within the wall of the descending thoracic aorta, consistent with a Stanford type B intramural hematoma (Fig. A). Axial contrast-enhanced CT scan performed 3 days earlier than Fig. 1 showed thickening of the descending thoracic aortic wall (Fig. B).

Notes

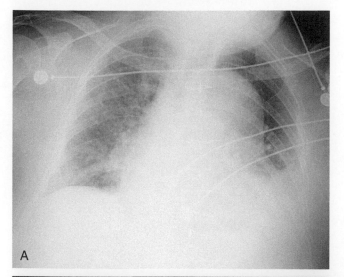

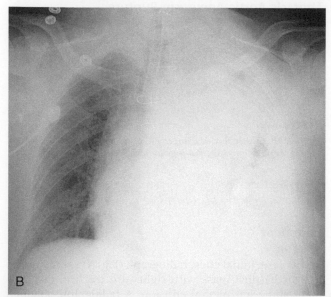

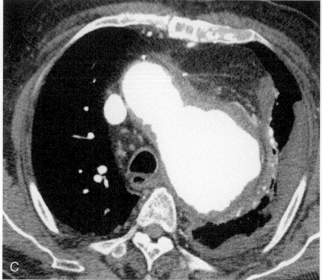

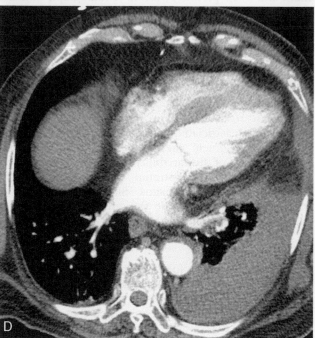

History: A 70-year-old woman suddenly becomes unresponsive.

1. What should be included in the differential diagnosis for Fig. A? (Choose all that apply.)
   A. Aortic aneurysm
   B. Enlarged main pulmonary artery
   C. Thymoma
   D. Sarcoidosis

2. What is the most likely diagnosis in this case?
   A. Intramural hematoma
   B. Ruptured aneurysm
   C. Aortic dissection
   D. Penetrating ulcer

3. Which of the following signs indicates contained or impending aortic rupture?
   A. "Draped aorta"
   B. "Oreo cookie"
   C. "Figure 3"
   D. "Intimal flap"

4. In which situation is earlier repair of a thoracic aortic aneurysm generally performed?
   A. Asymptomatic
   B. Emphysema
   C. Marfan syndrome
   D. Young patient

Thoracic Aortic Aneurysm Rupture

1. A, B, and C

2. B

3. A

4. C

Reference

Agarwal PP, Chughtai A, Matzinger FR, et al: Multidetector CT of thoracic aortic aneurysms, *Radiographics* 29(2):537-552, 2009.

Cross-Reference

Cardiac Imaging: The REQUISITES, ed 3, pp 405-408.

Comment

Imaging

In this case, initial chest radiograph (Fig. A) shows a large left mediastinal mass with rightward tracheal displacement and a left pleural effusion. A radiograph obtained 6 hours later (Fig. B) reveals interval intubation and near-complete left hemithorax opacification. Chest CT (Fig. C) shows a distal aortic arch aneurysm. There is a large amount of left pleural fluid with high density, consistent with hemothorax and aneurysm rupture (Figs. C and D).

Prognostic Signs

The main risk associated with a thoracic aortic aneurysm is rupture. Thoracic aneurysms should be monitored yearly because of the variability in growth rate. They can rupture into the mediastinum, pleural space, pericardium, airway, or esophagus. Signs of contained or impending rupture include the "draped aorta" sign or high-attenuation blood within mural thrombus.

Management

Surgical intervention for thoracic aortic aneurysms is recommended when the risk of rupture exceeds the risk of surgical intervention. Most surgeons repair asymptomatic ascending aortic aneurysms when they attain a size of 5.5 cm and descending aneurysms when they attain a size of 6.5 cm. Earlier intervention is recommended in patients with rapid growth of the aneurysm (>1 cm/year), in patients with symptoms from the aneurysm, and in patients with Marfan syndrome.

Notes

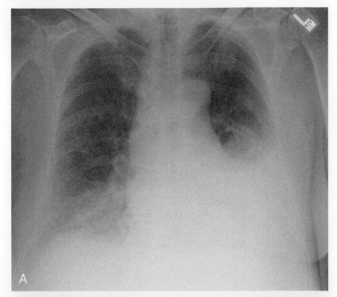

A

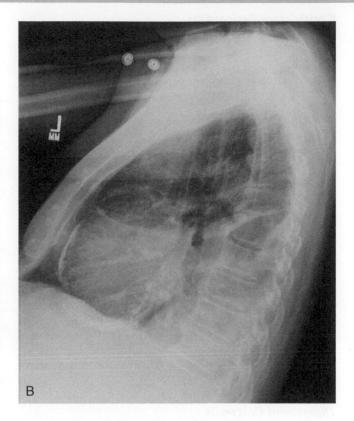

B

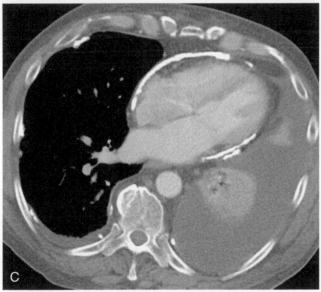

C

History: No patient history is available.

1. What should be included in the differential diagnosis? (Choose all that apply.)
   A. Tuberculosis infection
   B. Doxorubicin (Adriamycin) therapy
   C. Amyloidosis
   D. Uremia
   E. Radiation therapy

2. Which cardiac structure is calcified?
   A. Endocardium
   B. Epicardium
   C. Mitral anulus
   D. Pericardium

3. What is the most likely diagnosis if this patient presented with progressive dyspnea, ascites, and lower extremity edema?
   A. Constrictive pericarditis
   B. Restrictive cardiomyopathy
   C. Dilated cardiomyopathy
   D. Hypertrophic cardiomyopathy

4. What is the preferred treatment for this condition?
   A. Heart transplantation
   B. Pericardial stripping
   C. Medical management
   D. Ethanol ablation

Constrictive Pericarditis

1. A, D, and E

2. D

3. A

4. B

Reference

Wang ZJ, Reddy GP, Gotway MB, et al: CT and MR imaging of pericardial disease, *Radiographics* 23 Spec No:S167–S180, 2003.

Cross-Reference

Cardiac Imaging: The REQUISITES, ed 3, pp 269–276.

Comment

Imaging

Chest radiograph shows a large left pleural effusion and extensive pericardial calcification, best visualized on the lateral radiograph (Figs. A and B). Chest CT confirms these findings and shows bilateral calcified pleural plaques indicating asbestos exposure (Fig. C). Extensive pericardial calcification is diagnostic of constrictive pericarditis in the setting of constrictive or restrictive physiology.

Differential Diagnosis

Symptoms and signs of constrictive pericarditis are non-specific and include dyspnea, orthopnea, lower extremity edema, and ascites. CT and MRI are useful to differentiate constrictive pericarditis from restrictive cardiomyopathy. This distinction is important because treatments are vastly different. Constrictive pericarditis is treated surgically with pericardial stripping, whereas restrictive cardiomyopathy is managed medically or with heart transplantation. In patients with constrictive or restrictive physiology, ventricular filling is reduced leading to equalization of atrial and ventricular pressures. Echocardiography is unable to depict pericardial thickening accurately. Cross-sectional imaging findings of constrictive pericarditis include a pericardial thickness greater than or equal to 4 mm, pericardial calcification (Figs. B and C), and a diastolic septal bounce. Pericardial thickening may be diffuse or localized to the right heart or atrioventricular grooves.

Notes

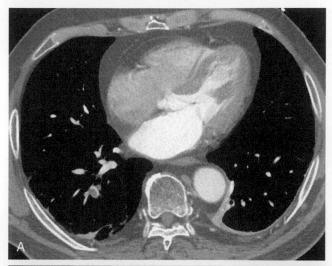

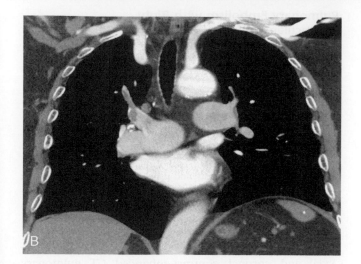

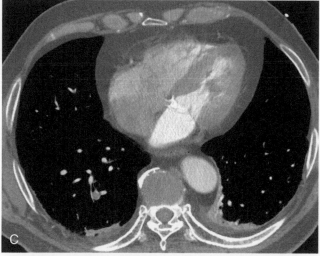

History: A patient presents with pleuritic chest pain and hypoxia.

1. Which of the following are risk factors for this diagnosis? (Choose all that apply.)
   A. Surgery 2 months ago
   B. Malignancy
   C. Paralysis
   D. Cigarette smoking

2. What cardiac finding is seen in Fig. B?
   A. Leftward bowing of interventricular septum
   B. Left atrial mass
   C. Pericardial effusion
   D. Left ventricular thrombus

3. What is the most likely cause of the cardiac finding in this patient with pulmonary embolism?
   A. Right ventricular strain
   B. Normal
   C. Right atrial thrombus
   D. Ventricular septal defect

4. Which of these findings indicates right heart strain in a patient with pulmonary embolism?
   A. Rightward bowing of interventricular septum
   B. Main pulmonary artery diameter greater than 20 mm
   C. Right ventricular-to-left ventricular (RV/LV) ratio greater than 1
   D. Right atrial enlargement

CASE 12

Pulmonary Embolism with Right Ventricular Strain

1. A, B, C, and D

2. A

3. A

4. C

Reference

Ghaye B, Ghuysen A, Bruyere PJ, et al: Can CT pulmonary angiography allow assessment of severity and prognosis in patients presenting with pulmonary embolism? What the radiologist needs to know, *Radiographics* 26(1):23-39, 2006; discussion 39-40.

Comment

Imaging

Axial and coronal contrast-enhanced CT pulmonary angiogram images (Figs. A-C) show multiple segmental and right upper lobar pulmonary emboli. Images of the heart show leftward bowing of the interventricular septum and an elevated RV/LV ratio measuring 1.2. This elevated ratio indicates right heart strain.

Prognostic Indicators

Pulmonary embolism remains a common clinical problem despite advances in thromboembolism prophylaxis. Two large multicenter trials found a significantly higher mortality in patients presenting with hemodynamic instability (50% to 58% mortality compared with 8% to 15% mortality in hemodynamically stable patients). Several CT findings have been shown to be predictive of right heart strain and impending hemodynamic instability. Commenting on these CT findings in an imaging report allows the clinician to initiate appropriate management and patient monitoring. The most sensitive and specific imaging sign is an abnormal RV/LV ratio greater than 1 (Figs. A and C). This ratio compares the short-axis diameters of the right ventricle and left ventricle. The right ventricular and left ventricular short axis diameters are measured on axial images at the respective levels of the tricuspid and mitral valves. The largest inner-to-inner diameter of the right ventricle and left ventricle is taken to measure the short-axis diameter. In normal patients, the left ventricular short axis is always larger than the right ventricular short axis, and the RV/LV ratio is less than 1. A RV/LV ratio greater than 1 is a highly sensitive and specific sign of right ventricular strain. An abnormal RV/LV ratio is predictive of higher patient mortality and a 3.6 times higher rate of intensive care unit admission. Other signs of right heart strain include leftward interventricular septal shift and a main pulmonary arterial diameter greater than 30 mm.

Notes

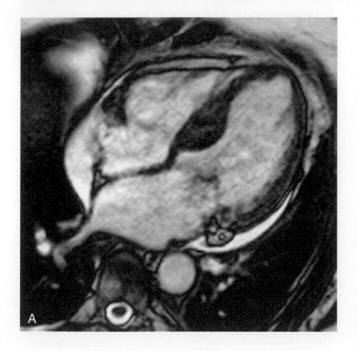

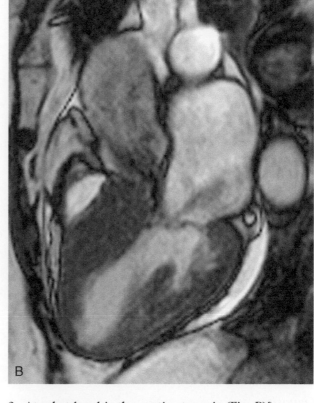

History: No patient history is available.

1. What should be included in the differential diagnosis? (Choose all that apply.)
   A. Amyloidosis
   B. Bicuspid aortic valve
   C. Mitral valve prolapse
   D. Hypertrophic cardiomyopathy (HCM)
   E. Fabry disease

2. What is the main myocardial finding?
   A. Delayed enhancement
   B. Myocardial mass
   C. Lipomatous hypertrophy
   D. Basal interventricular septal hypertrophy

3. At what level is the aortic stenosis (Fig. B)?
   A. Subaortic
   B. Valvular
   C. Supravalvular
   D. No evidence of aortic stenosis

4. What is the most common variant of HCM?
   A. Concentric
   B. Apical
   C. Asymmetric septal
   D. Masslike

Asymmetric Septal Hypertrophy Variant of Hypertrophic Cardiomyopathy

1. D and E

2. D

3. A

4. C

Reference

Chun EJ, Choi SI, Jin KN, et al: Hypertrophic cardiomyopathy: assessment with MR imaging and multidetector CT, *Radiographics* 30(5):1309-1328, 2010.

Cross-Reference

Cardiac Imaging: The REQUISITES, ed 3, pp 284-288.

Comment

Imaging

Cine steady-state free precession (SSFP) four-chamber view shows basal interventricular septal hypertrophy (Fig. A). Cine SSFP left ventricular outflow tract view shows flow void jets of mitral regurgitation and aortic stenosis (Fig. B). These findings are consistent with the asymmetric form of HCM. This diagnosis should be made only in the absence of a systemic condition that could cause myocardial hypertrophy.

Diagnosis

HCM is an inherited cardiomyopathy characterized histologically by myocyte disarray and interstitial fibrosis. These histologic findings lead to an increased risk for fatal arrhythmia and sudden cardiac death. Echocardiography is the standard screening modality for patients suspected to have HCM. MRI is used in difficult cases, in unusual patterns of HCM, and in patients who are candidates for invasive therapy. MRI is superior in assessing left ventricular function and in determining the overall risk for sudden cardiac death. This case shows the most common HCM phenotype, asymmetric septal hypertrophy. Asymmetric HCM is diagnosed when a portion of the septum measures 15 mm or more at end-diastole. There are two clinically important subtypes of asymmetric HCM—obstructive and nonobstructive forms. The obstructive form is characterized by dynamic left ventricular outflow obstruction caused by the hypertrophied septum or systolic anterior motion of the mitral valve. Patients with obstructive HCM should be evaluated for possible intervention using septal alcohol ablation or surgical myectomy.

Prognostic Indicators

MRI is a useful prognostic indicator for risk of sudden cardiac death. Specific imaging findings that indicate an increased risk include the following:

1. Left ventricular wall thickness measuring greater than 30 mm

2. Left ventricular outflow tract pressure gradient greater than 30 mmHg at rest or greater than 50 mm Hg with provocative maneuvers as depicted on velocity-encoded cine phase contrast MRI

3. Fibrosis indicated by late gadolinium enhancement within myocardium in a nonvascular distribution

4. Left ventricular dilation with reduced ejection fraction (so-called burned-out HCM)

5. Perfusion defects

Notes

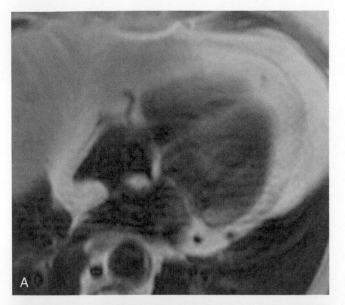

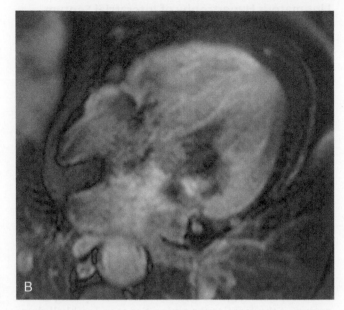

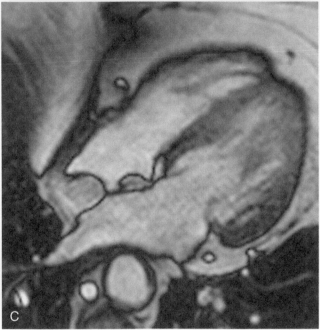

History: A patient has a mass seen on echocardiography.

1. What should be included in the differential diagnosis for a precontrast T1 hyperintense cardiac mass? (Choose all that apply.)
   A. Lipoma
   B. Lipomatous hypertrophy of the interatrial septum
   C. Breast cancer metastasis
   D. Melanoma metastasis
   E. Myxoma

2. What is the most common presentation for this entity?
   A. Arrhythmia
   B. Thromboembolism
   C. Asymptomatic
   D. Superior vena cava obstruction

3. What is the composition of this lesion?
   A. Proteinaceous fluid
   B. Intracellular methemoglobin
   C. Melanin
   D. Fat

4. What is the appropriate management in an asymptomatic patient?
   A. Do nothing
   B. Surgical resection
   C. CT with contrast medium
   D. Arrhythmia prophylaxis

CASE 14

Lipomatous Hypertrophy of Interatrial Septum

1. A, B, and D

2. C

3. D

4. A

Reference

Gaerte SC, Meyer CA, Winer-Muram HT, et al: Fat-containing lesions of the chest, *Radiographics* 22 Spec No:S61–S78, 2002.

Cross-Reference

Cardiac Imaging: The REQUISITES, ed 3, pp 281–282.

Comment

Imaging

Axial black blood T1-weighted images without and with fat suppression show a fat density mass within the interatrial septum (Figs. A and B). There is sparing in the region of the fossa ovalis giving rise to a dumbbell shape of the lesion (Fig. C). These features are diagnostic of lipomatous hypertrophy of the interatrial septum.

Diagnosis

Lipomatous hypertrophy of the interatrial septum is a benign condition that is usually incidentally discovered on imaging performed for other reasons. It represents an abnormal deposition of fat within the atrial septum that is greater than 2 cm in transverse dimension. It is more common in older women and obese patients. Echocardiography occasionally mistakes this entity for a cardiac mass. Diagnosis is easily made with either CT or MRI. The location and lesion shape differentiate it from cardiac lipoma and physiologic myocardial fat. Rarely, patients are symptomatic and present with arrhythmia.

Notes

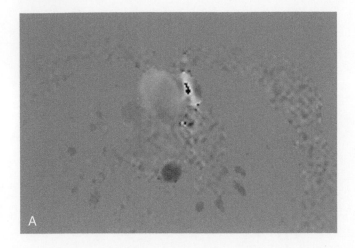

A

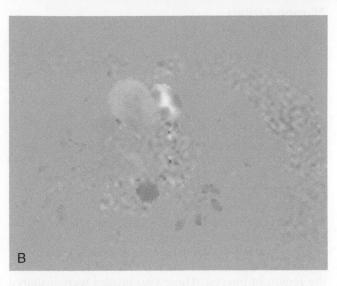

B

History: A patient undergoes imaging for aortic stenosis quantification.

1. Which of the following are considered MRI artifacts? (Choose all that apply.)
   A. Banding
   B. Radiofrequency
   C. Aliasing
   D. Wraparound
   E. Dark rim

2. What imaging sequence is shown?
   A. Cine steady-state free precession (SSFP)
   B. Velocity-encoded cine phase contrast MRI
   C. Late gadolinium enhancement
   D. Black blood

3. Why is this sequence performed in a patient with aortic valve stenosis?
   A. Quantification
   B. Detect stenosis
   C. Anatomic detail
   D. Assess the effect on myocardium

4. What is the name of the imaging artifact in Fig. A?
   A. Radiofrequency
   B. Breathing
   C. Ghost artifact
   D. Aliasing

CASE 15

Aliasing Artifact

1. A, B, C, D, and E

2. B

3. A

4. D

Reference

Saremi F, Grizzard JD, Kim RJ: Optimizing cardiac MR imaging: practical remedies for artifacts, *Radiographics* 28(4):1161–1187, 2008.

Comment

Imaging Appearance

Two images from velocity-encoded cine phase contrast MRI demonstrate the imaging artifact of aliasing (Figs. A and B). Aliasing occurs when the encoded velocity set by the user is not higher than the actual velocity across the region of interest. These two images were acquired for quantification of known aortic stenosis. Cranial flow is depicted as white signal, and caudal flow is depicted as black signal. In the first image, the velocity-encoded gradient was set at 300 cm/s. There is black signal surrounded by white signal within the ascending aorta (Fig. A). This is physically impossible, and the imaging appearance is an aliasing artifact (wraparound or apparent velocity reversal). In the second image, the velocity-encoded gradient was increased to 350 cm/s, and the aliasing disappeared (Fig. B). The maximum velocity-encoded gradient should ideally be selected to exceed slightly the expected peak velocity.

Notes

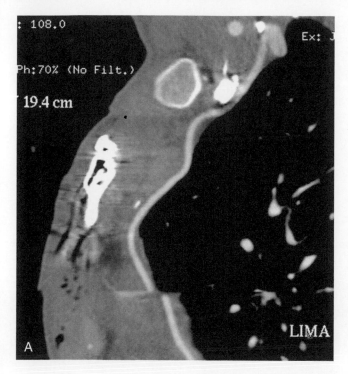

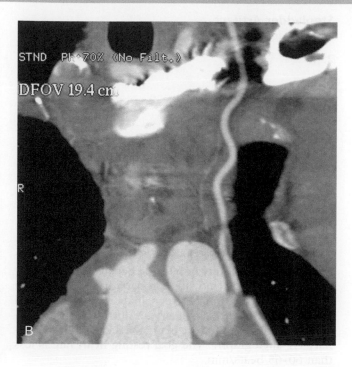

History: A patient presents with chest pain; there is concern for graft occlusion.

1. Which of the following are artifacts seen on CT angiography? (Choose all that apply.)
   A. Stepladder
   B. Ghosting
   C. Beam hardening
   D. Motion blur

2. What imaging artifact is shown?
   A. Stepladder artifact
   B. Banding
   C. Beam hardening from air bubble
   D. Motion blur

3. What imaging plane is shown?
   A. Coronal
   B. Sagittal
   C. Curved multiplanar reformat
   D. Axial

4. What is the likely cause of the stepladder artifact?
   A. High heart rate
   B. Patient motion
   C. Photon loss or "starvation"
   D. Faulty detector

Stepladder Artifact

1. A, C, and D

2. A

3. C

4. B

Reference

Choi HS, Choi BW, Choe KO, et al: Pitfalls, artifacts, and remedies in multi-detector row CT coronary angiography, *Radiographics* 24(3):787–800, 2004.

Comment

Causes

Motion-related artifacts fall into two categories: blurring or stepladder artifact. The right coronary artery is the most susceptible artery to blurring because it is the most mobile and rapidly moving coronary artery. There is a significant correlation between higher heart rates and poorer image quality secondary to blurring. This correlation forms the basis for use of beta blockade before coronary CT angiography. The goal resting heart rate is less than 60–65 beats/min.

Types of Stepladder Artifact

Stepladder artifact occurs whenever there is patient movement, respiration, or a varying heart rate. This artifact is identified by recognizing an abrupt linear offset of data (Figs. A and B). When stepladder artifact involves the anterior chest wall, it is due to respiration or patient movement and not a varying heart rate. Cardiac-related stepladder artifact can be reduced by minimizing the heart rate through the use of beta blockers and by choosing the appropriate reconstruction window within the R-R interval. Respiratory-related artifact or artifact related to voluntary motion is often easily prevented with careful patient instructions before imaging and oxygen for dyspneic patients.

Notes

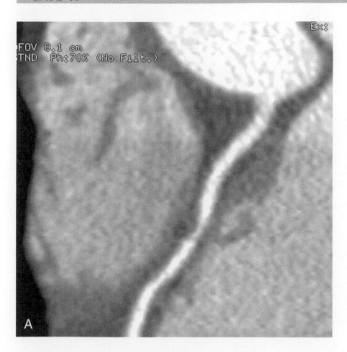

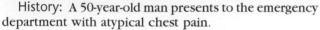

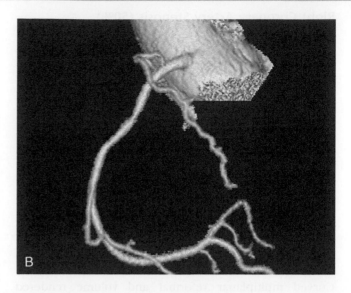

History: A 50-year-old man presents to the emergency department with atypical chest pain.

1. What should be included in the differential diagnosis? (Choose all that apply.)
   A. Artifactual narrowing of coronary artery
   B. Coronary artery dissection
   C. Noncalcified plaque
   D. Calcified plaque

2. What degree of coronary arterial narrowing is considered a positive CT angiography result?
   A. 0%
   B. 15%
   C. 35%
   D. 50%

3. What is the finding in the right coronary artery?
   A. Normal
   B. 20% narrowing
   C. 50% narrowing
   D. Dissection

4. What is the best next step for management of this patient with a 50% narrowing?
   A. Coronary stent
   B. Medical management
   C. Coronary artery bypass graft surgery
   D. Coronary angiography

Right Coronary Artery Stenosis (50%)

1. C

2. D

3. C

4. D

Reference

Townsend JC, Gregg D IV: Cardiac computed tomography and magnetic resonance imaging: the clinical use from a cardiologist's perspective, *J Thorac Imaging* 25(3):194–203, 2010.

Cross-Reference

Cardiac Imaging: The REQUISITES, ed 3, pp 248–261.

Comment

Imaging

Curved multiplanar reformat and volume rendered images show a focal stenosis with diameter reduction of approximately 50% in the proximal right coronary artery (Figs. A and B). The narrowing consists of noncalcified plaque without calcification.

Further Evaluation

The clinical utility of CT angiography of the coronary arteries is highly dependent on the patient population studied. The diagnostic value of CT angiography is greatest in patients with a low pretest probability of disease and is lowest in patients with a high pretest probability of disease. In other words, CT angiography has a high negative predictive value for excluding disease in patients with a low or intermediate pretest probability of coronary artery disease. Patients with a negative test do not need further evaluation for coronary disease. In this case, the test is positive (≥50% narrowing) and the patient needs a coronary angiogram to confirm the presence of significant disease. Coronary catheterization confirmed right coronary artery stenosis with a 60% diameter reduction, and this was successfully treated with a stent.

Patient Selection

The ideal patient to undergo CT angiography of the coronary arteries is a patient with a low or intermediate pretest probability of coronary artery disease. CT angiography is not indicated in patients with typical findings of coronary artery disease or in patients with a high pretest likelihood of disease (i.e., ECG changes suggestive of ischemia or laboratory evidence of myocardial injury). CT angiography of the coronary arteries is also not indicated in patients suspected to have another disease (i.e., pneumonia, pneumothorax, or pulmonary embolism).

Notes

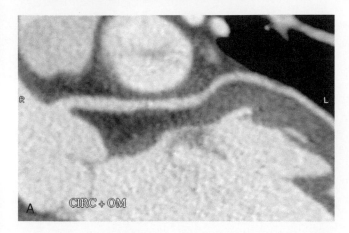

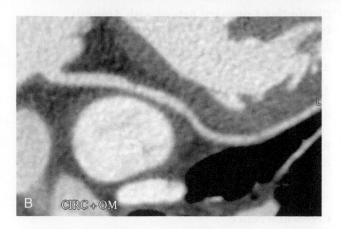

History: A 40-year-old man presents with atypical chest pain.

1. Which of the following would require coronary catheterization after coronary CT angiography? (Choose all that apply.)
   A. 40% stenosis of left anterior descending coronary artery
   B. 20% stenosis of left anterior descending coronary artery
   C. 60% stenosis of left anterior descending coronary artery
   D. 70% stenosis of left anterior descending coronary artery

2. What is the major benefit of coronary CT angiography in the evaluation of a low-risk patient with chest pain?
   A. High negative predictive value
   B. High positive predictive value
   C. High specificity
   D. High accuracy

3. What is the finding in the left circumflex coronary artery?
   A. Less than 50% narrowing by noncalcified plaque
   B. Less than 50% narrowing by calcified plaque
   C. Greater than 50% narrowing by noncalcified plaque
   D. Greater than 50% narrowing by calcified plaque

4. What is the most appropriate recommendation for this patient?
   A. Coronary stent
   B. Medical management
   C. Coronary artery bypass graft surgery
   D. Coronary angiography

CASE 18

Circumflex Coronary Artery with Stenosis (<50%)

1. C and D

2. A

3. A

4. B

Reference

Zimmet JM, Miller JM: Coronary artery CTA: imaging of atherosclerosis in the coronary arteries and reporting of coronary artery CTA findings, *Tech Vasc Interv Radiol* 9(4):218-226, 2006.

Cross-Reference

Cardiac Imaging: The REQUISITES, ed 3, pp 248-261.

Comment

Imaging

Two multiplanar reformatted images show a short segment stenosis with 20% to 30% diameter reduction in the proximal left circumflex coronary artery. The plaque is eccentric and noncalcified (Figs. A and B).

Diagnosis

The main value of CT angiography is excluding significant coronary artery disease in patients presenting with chest pain who are deemed to have a low or intermediate risk of having had a coronary event. CT angiography is able to exclude disease because of its high negative predictive value in this specific patient population. The degree of vessel stenosis is determined by comparing the luminal diameter at the site of greatest narrowing with the luminal diameter of the most proximal normal segment of coronary artery. A positive CT angiography result is defined as a stenosis with luminal diameter reduction greater than or equal to 50%. Patients with a positive examination must be evaluated further with catheter angiography to confirm and define the abnormality further and potentially to treat the culprit lesion.

Notes

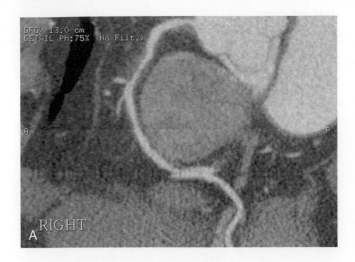

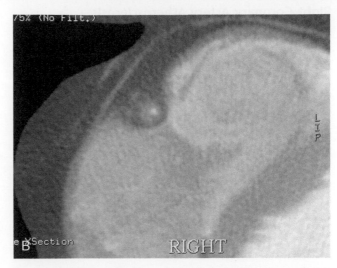

History: A 35-year-old man presents with atypical chest pain.

1. What medications are often used before performing this examination? (Choose all that apply.)
   A. Oral beta blocker
   B. Amiodarone
   C. Intravenous beta blocker
   D. Nitroglycerin
   E. Angiotensin-converting enzyme inhibitor

2. Which coronary artery is most affected by cardiac motion?
   A. Left circumflex
   B. Left anterior descending
   C. Left main
   D. Right

3. What is the finding in the right coronary artery?
   A. Normal
   B. Myocardial bridge with stenosis
   C. Greater than 50% narrowing
   D. Less than 50% narrowing

4. Assuming the other coronary arteries were normal, what is the next best step in management?
   A. Diagnostic catheter angiogram
   B. Coronary artery bypass graft surgery
   C. Coronary stent
   D. Medical management

CASE 19

Right Coronary Artery Atherosclerosis Causing 60% Narrowing

1. A, C, and D

2. D

3. C

4. A

Reference

Kerl JM, Hofmann LK, Thilo C, et al: Coronary CTA: image acquisition and interpretation, *J Thorac Imaging* 22(1):22-34, 2007.

Cross-Reference

Cardiac Imaging: The REQUISITES, ed 3, pp 248-261.

Comment

Imaging

A multiplanar reformatted image from CT angiography shows a circumferential, focal stenosis of the proximal right coronary artery composed entirely of noncalcified plaque (Fig. A). The degree of narrowing is best appreciated on the short-axis image; the stenosis measures approximately 60% (Fig. B).

Benefits of CT Angiography

The main benefit of CT angiography is that it excludes coronary artery disease in patients presenting with chest pain. Patients with ST segment elevation, typical angina, and elevated cardiac enzymes do not require CT angiography but rather undergo emergent revascularization therapy. CT angiography is best used as a test in patients with a low or intermediate pretest probability of disease. In these patients, CT angiography has a low number of false-positive results and essentially no false-negative results. It has been shown to reduce overall cost and length of hospital stay in this patient subgroup.

Heart Rate Control

Patient preparation is an important aspect of imaging that must not be overlooked. A target heart rate less than 65 to 70 beats/min is desired to achieve motion-free images. Either intravenous or oral beta blockers may be given to achieve a target heart rate. When the patient is on the scanner table, 5 mg of intravenous metoprolol may be given. This dose can be repeated for a total dose of 15 to 25 mg. Alternatively, oral metoprolol may be given. A dose of 50 to 100 mg may be given the night before the scan, with an additional dose 30 to 60 minutes before starting the CT angiography scan. A third dose may be given if adequate rate control is not achieved. A drawback of oral dosing is the added time required to achieve adequate drug levels.

Vasodilators

Nitroglycerin is commonly administered before CT angiography at a dose of 300 to 600 micrograms sublingually 2 minutes before starting the scan. Nitroglycerin vasodilates the coronary arteries, which leads to better visualization of the arteries and may reduce coronary spasm, which is more prevalent in younger patients.

Notes

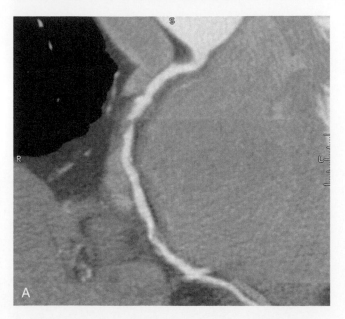

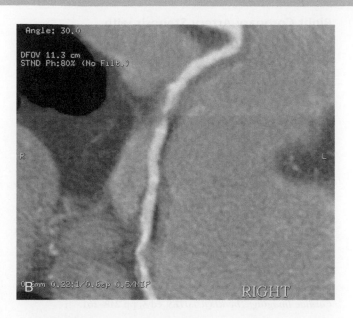

History: A 63-year-old man presents to the emergency department with atypical chest pain.

1. Which of the following are considered significant limitations for CT angiography of the coronary arteries? (Choose all that apply.)
   A. Motion artifact
   B. Blooming artifact
   C. Contrast agent allergy
   D. Radiation

2. What is the finding in the right coronary artery?
   A. High-grade stenosis (>70%)
   B. 50% stenosis
   C. 30% stenosis
   D. Normal

3. What is the next best step in management assuming the other coronary arteries were normal?
   A. Do nothing
   B. Medical management
   C. Diagnostic catheter angiogram
   D. Stent placement

4. What is the gold standard for characterization of coronary plaque?
   A. CT angiography
   B. MRI
   C. Intravascular ultrasound
   D. Coronary angiography

CASE 20

Right Coronary Artery Stenosis with Approximately 80% Narrowing

1. A, B, C, and D

2. A

3. C

4. C

References

Sundaram B, Patel S, Agarwal P, et al: Anatomy and terminology for the interpretation and reporting of cardiac MDCT: part 2, CT angiography, cardiac function assessment, and noncoronary and extracardiac findings, *AJR Am J Roentgenol* 192(3):584-598, 2009.🕮

Sundaram B, Patel S, Bogot N, et al: Anatomy and terminology for the interpretation and reporting of cardiac MDCT: part 1, structured report, coronary calcium screening, and coronary artery anatomy, *AJR Am J Roentgenol* 192(3):574-583, 2009.🕮

Cross-Reference

Cardiac Imaging: The REQUISITES, ed 3, pp 248-261.

Comment

Imaging

This patient presented to the emergency department with atypical chest pain and was deemed to be at low to intermediate risk for coronary artery disease. The patient was triaged with triple rule-out CT angiography of the thorax to exclude coronary artery disease, pulmonary embolism, and aortic dissection. This examination revealed no pulmonary embolism or aortic dissection. Two multiplanar reformatted images of the right coronary artery showed a focal high-grade stenosis (approximately 80%) composed entirely of noncalcified plaque (Figs. A and B). Subsequently, the patient underwent diagnostic cardiac catheterization, which confirmed right coronary artery stenosis. A successful balloon angioplasty with stent placement was performed with resolution of the patient's symptoms.

Utility

Millions of people present to the emergency department annually with the complaint of chest pain. Only 20% to 25% of these patients are found to have a coronary etiology of their pain at the time of discharge. CT angiography can be used to triage these patients rapidly and diagnose important extracardiac causes of chest pain. It is ideally used in patients with a low or intermediate pretest probability of disease based on their risk factors and clinical presentation. A positive examination (i.e., coronary stenosis ≥50%) must be confirmed with diagnostic catheterization, whereas a negative examination (i.e., any stenosis <50%) needs no further testing because the lesion is unlikely to be the cause of the patient's chest pain.

Notes

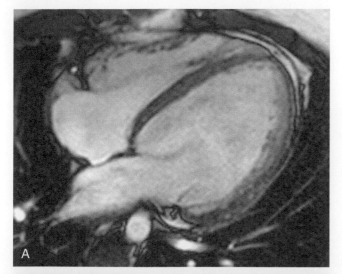

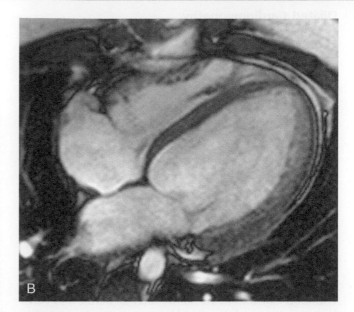

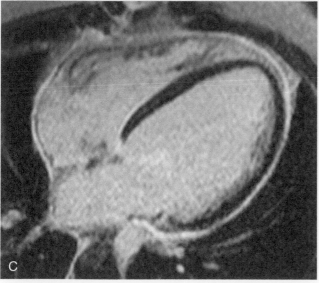

History: A 29-year-old man presents with progressive dyspnea on exertion and profound fatigue.

1. What are potential causes of this entity? (Choose all that apply.)
   A. Idiopathic
   B. Alcohol
   C. Anthracyclines
   D. Infection
   E. Duchenne muscular dystrophy

2. What is the finding on the precontrast bright blood sequences? (Fig. A was obtained at end-diastole, and Fig. B was obtained at end-systole.)
   A. Dilated cardiac chambers and low ejection fraction
   B. Pericardial thickening
   C. Concentric myocardial hypertrophy
   D. Spin dephasing flow void artifact

3. What is the most common cause of congestive heart failure?
   A. Dilated cardiomyopathy
   B. Ischemic cardiomyopathy
   C. Valvular heart disease
   D. Myocarditis

4. What is the likely cause of this patient's congestive heart failure?
   A. Amyloidosis
   B. Valvular heart disease
   C. Ischemic cardiomyopathy
   D. Nonischemic dilated cardiomyopathy

Dilated Cardiomyopathy

1. A, B, C, D, and E

2. A

3. B

4. D

Reference

Sparrow PJ, Merchant N, Provost YL, et al: CT and MR imaging findings in patients with acquired heart disease at risk for sudden cardiac death, *Radiographics* 29(3):805-823, 2009.

Cross-Reference

Cardiac Imaging: The REQUISITES, ed 3, pp 87-88, 284-286.

Comment

Overview

Nonischemic dilated cardiomyopathy is the third most common cause of heart failure after ischemic and valvular heart disease. It is caused by various insults, including alcohol, medications, infections, and various neuromuscular syndromes. Frequently, it is familial or idiopathic. Histologically, there is loss of myocytes with progressive deposition of interstitial fibrosis leading to impaired ventricular contraction.

Imaging

Cine steady-state free precession (SSFP) four-chamber view images show dilation of all four cardiac chambers (Figs. A and B). There is a severely reduced ejection fraction, which was measured at 14%. Late gadolinium enhancement is noted in the midportion of the interventricular septum (Fig. C).

Presentation

Patients usually present with congestive heart failure, arrhythmias, or cardiac thromboembolism secondary to ventricular hypocontractility. Imaging findings include ventricular dilation and impaired myocardial contractility with reduction in ejection fraction. Midmyocardial late gadolinium enhancement is seen in 12% to 35% of patients (Fig. C).

Prognosis and Treatment

Patient mortality is due to heart failure or sudden cardiac death from ventricular arrhythmia. Specific imaging risk factors that convey an increased risk for sudden cardiac death include a reduced left ventricular ejection fraction (<35%) and late gadolinium myocardial enhancement (affecting 25% to 75% of the myocardial wall). Treatment is symptomatic management of heart failure. Heart transplantation is the definitive therapy.

Notes

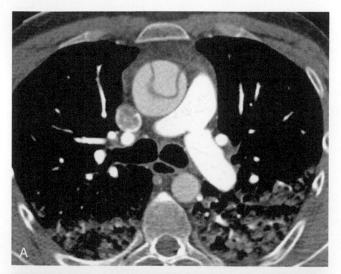

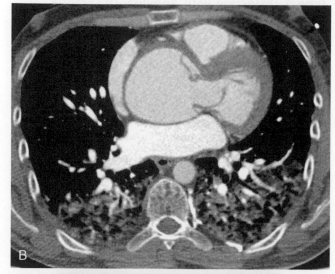

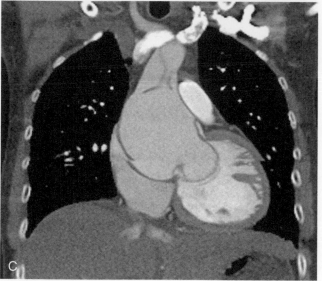

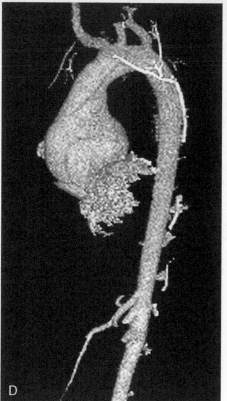

History: A 34-year-old man presents with shortness of breath, dizziness, and chest pain.

1. What are life-threatening complications of this disease? (Choose all that apply.)
   A. Tamponade
   B. Stroke
   C. Myocardial infarction
   D. Aortic rupture

2. What is the term used to describe the appearance of this ascending aorta?
   A. Annuloaortic ectasia
   B. Sinus of Valsalva aneurysm
   C. Diverticulum of Kommerell
   D. Saccular aneurysm

3. Which of the following conditions is most commonly associated with annuloaortic ectasia?
   A. Ehlers-Danlos syndrome
   B. Turner syndrome
   C. Marfan syndrome
   D. Kawasaki syndrome

4. Which complication of annuloaortic ectasia has occurred in this patient?
   A. Aortic valve stenosis
   B. Aortic rupture
   C. Tamponade
   D. Aortic dissection

45

Type A Dissection with Annuloaortic Ectasia

1. A, B, C, and D

2. A

3. C

4. D

Reference

Ha HI, Seo JB, Lee SH, et al: Imaging of Marfan syndrome: multisystemic manifestations, *Radiographics* 27(4):989–1004, 2007.

Cross-Reference

Cardiac Imaging: The REQUISITES, ed 3, pp 378-391.

Comment

Imaging

Axial and coronal images from prospectively gated CT angiography of the thoracic aorta show a Stanford type A aortic dissection (Figs. A-C). The intimal flap is prolapsed through the aortic valve causing aortic regurgitation (Figs. B and C). The ascending aorta is shaped like a pear or tulip bulb (Figs. C and D), which is consistent with annuloaortic ectasia. Annuloaortic ectasia is most commonly seen in Marfan syndrome but can occur in other connective tissue diseases such as Ehlers-Danlos syndrome.

Complications

Annuloaortic ectasia occurs secondary to cystic medial necrosis, which may be idiopathic or associated with Marfan syndrome or Ehlers-Danlos syndrome. Three main complications of this condition include aortic rupture, aortic regurgitation, and aortic dissection. Early operative repair of a thoracic aortic aneurysm is performed when the diameter reaches 5 cm in patients with Marfan syndrome because of the high risk of rupture.

Notes

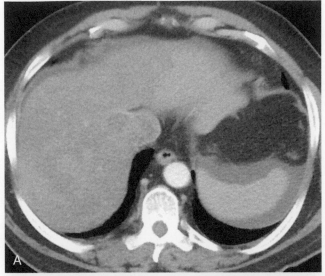

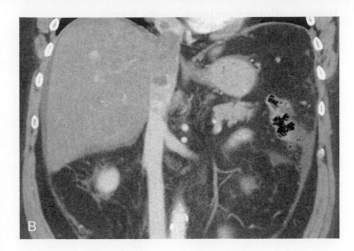

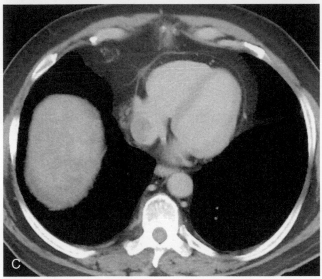

History: A 65-year-old man presents with a 1-month history of abdominal pain.

1. What tumors can invade the inferior vena cava (IVC)? (Choose all that apply.)
   A. Adrenocortical carcinoma
   B. Hepatocellular carcinoma (HCC)
   C. Renal cell carcinoma
   D. Lung carcinoma

2. What is the cardiac finding?
   A. Primary benign tumor
   B. Metastatic tumor
   C. Primary malignant tumor
   D. Bland thrombus

3. What is the source of tumor thrombus?
   A. Adrenocortical carcinoma
   B. HCC
   C. Renal cell carcinoma
   D. Sarcoma

4. Which of the following is characteristic of a malignant cardiac mass?
   A. Well-circumscribed
   B. Infiltrative
   C. Involves one chamber
   D. No contrast enhancement

CASE 23

Hepatocellular Carcinoma with Tumor Thrombus Extending to Right Atrium

1. A, B, C, and D

2. B

3. B

4. B

Reference

Dedeilias P, Nenekidis I, Koukis I, et al: Acute heart failure caused by a giant hepatocellular metastatic tumor of the right atrium, *J Cardio-thorac Surg* 6:102, 2011.

Cross-Reference

Cardiac Imaging: The REQUISITES, ed 3, pp 277–278.

Comment

Imaging

Multiple images from a contrast-enhanced CT scan of the abdomen show a heterogeneously enhancing filling defect expanding the middle hepatic vein and IVC (Figs. A and B). The filling defect extends superiorly into the right atrium (Fig. C). These imaging findings are most consistent with tumor thrombus from HCC. Patients with HCC uncommonly present with metastatic disease (approximately 5%).

Overview

Invasion of the IVC and right atrium by tumor is uncommon. The three most common tumors to invade the IVC and right atrium are HCC, renal cell carcinoma, and adrenocortical carcinoma. Cardiac metastases secondary to HCC occur in 3% of all patients. Prompt diagnosis is important because tumor within the right atrium can cause congestive heart failure and sudden cardiac death. Surgical resection is palliative but rarely curative.

Notes

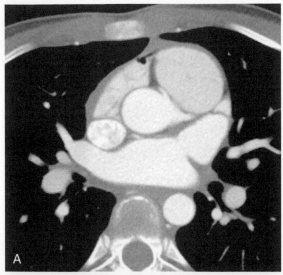

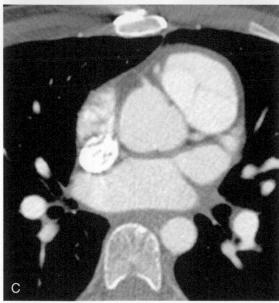

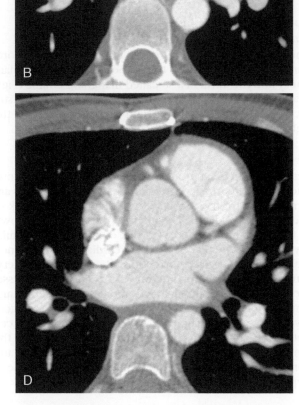

History: A 14-year-old girl presents for CT angiography after an echocardiogram showed an anomalous origin of the right coronary artery.

1. What are potential paths of an anomalous coronary artery? (Choose all that apply.)
   A. Retroaortic
   B. Prepulmonic
   C. Septal
   D. Interarterial

2. Which of the following best characterizes the course of the right coronary artery?
   A. Retroaortic
   B. Prepulmonic
   C. Septal
   D. Interarterial

3. If this patient had inferior myocardial ischemia on stress testing, what would be the best next step in management?
   A. Surgery
   B. Stenting
   C. Beta-blocker therapy
   D. No therapy needed

4. What has occurred between Figs. A and B and Figs. C and D?
   A. Stenting
   B. Reimplantation
   C. Bypass graft
   D. Angioplasty

Anomalous Right Coronary Artery with Interarterial Course

1. A, B, C, and D

2. D

3. A

4. B

Reference

Young PM, Gerber TC, Williamson EE, et al: Cardiac imaging: part 2, normal, variant, and anomalous configurations of the coronary vasculature, *AJR Am J Roentgenol* 197(4):816–826, 2011.

Cross-Reference

Cardiac Imaging: The REQUISITES, ed 3, pp 225–228.

Comment

Imaging

The right coronary artery originates from the left coronary sinus of Valsalva and travels between the pulmonary artery and the aorta in a so-called malignant course (Figs. A and B). This patient was treated successfully with surgical reimplantation of the right coronary artery to the right coronary cusp (Figs. C and D).

Overview

Ectopic origin of a coronary artery is the most frequently encountered coronary artery anomaly. Certain forms are benign and are not associated with an increased risk of sudden cardiac death. The interarterial course, as shown in this case, has an increased risk of angina, arrhythmia, myocardial ischemia, and sudden cardiac death. It generally requires surgical correction. Bypass graft surgery, unroofing, and reimplantation of the anomalous vessel are the available surgical options at the present time. This patient was treated with reimplantation surgery given her age at diagnosis. Coronary angiography can detect an anomalous vessel but cannot identify the course and relationship to the pulmonary artery and aorta. CT angiography guides management because it depicts the course of the vessel.

Notes

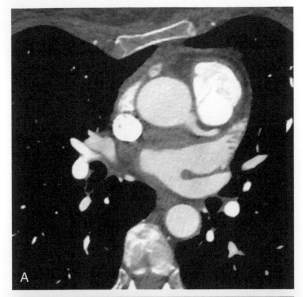

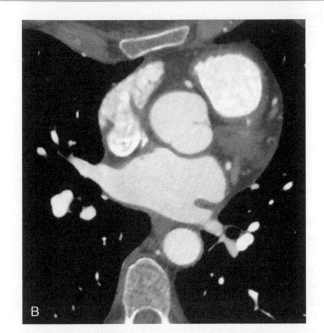

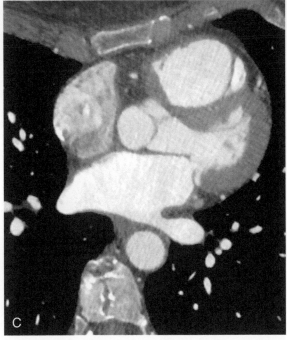

History: A 40-year-old man presents to the emergency department with atypical chest pain.

1. What vessels lie in the left atrioventricular groove? (Choose all that apply.)
   A. Right coronary artery (RCA)
   B. Posterior descending coronary artery
   C. Left circumflex
   D. Great cardiac vein
   E. Small cardiac vein

2. Which coronary artery has diagonal and septal perforator branches?
   A. Right
   B. Left main
   C. Left anterior descending
   D. Left circumflex

3. Which coronary artery lies in the inferior interventricular groove?
   A. Left anterior descending
   B. Posterior descending
   C. Left circumflex
   D. Right

4. Which coronary artery travels in the right atrioventricular groove?
   A. Right
   B. Left main
   C. Left circumflex
   D. Left anterior descending

CASE 25

Normal Coronary Artery Anatomy on CT Angiography

1. C and D

2. C

3. B

4. A

Reference

Young PM, Gerber TC, Williamson EE, et al: Cardiac imaging: part 2, normal, variant, and anomalous configurations of the coronary vasculature, *AJR Am J Roentgenol* 197(4):816-826, 2011.

Cross-Reference

Cardiac Imaging: The REQUISITES, ed 3, pp 110-115.

Comment

Imaging

This case illustrates normal coronary artery anatomy (Figs. A-C). The arteries are named according to where the blood flow goes (i.e., the RCA supplies the morphologic right ventricle).

Right Coronary Artery

The RCA originates from the right sinus of Valsalva and travels in the right atrioventricular groove. Its first branch, the conus branch, arises from the RCA in 50% of patients and supplies the right ventricular outflow tract. Other early branches of the RCA include the sinoatrial nodal and atrioventricular nodal arteries. The largest branches of the RCA are the acute marginal arteries, which supply the free wall of the right ventricle. The RCA is "dominant" in most patients (approximately 70-85%), supplying the inferior left ventricular myocardium and septum through the posterior descending coronary artery and posterolateral left ventricular branch.

Left Coronary Artery System

The left main coronary artery originates from the left sinus of Valsalva and is usually about 1 cm in length. It quickly divides into the left anterior descending and left circumflex coronary arteries. In 15% of patients, there is a trifurcation with the ramus intermedius being the named middle branch. The left circumflex coronary artery travels in the left atrioventricular groove and supplies the left ventricular free wall through obtuse marginal branches. The left circumflex coronary artery is dominant in about 10% of patients where it supplies the inferior wall of the left ventricle. Approximately 15% to 20% of patients have codominance of the RCA and left circumflex arteries. The left anterior descending coronary artery lies in the interventricular groove and gives off septal branches that supply the interventricular septum and diagonal branches that supply the anterior left ventricular wall.

Notes

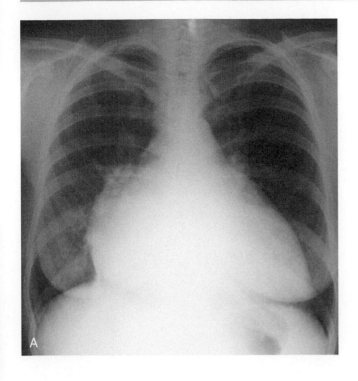

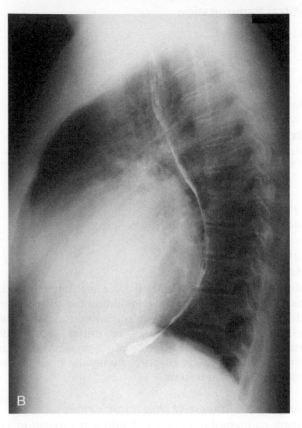

History: A patient presents with dyspnea on exertion.

1. What cardiac chambers are enlarged? (Choose all that apply.)
   A. Left atrium
   B. Left ventricle
   C. Right atrium
   D. Right ventricle

2. What is the most likely diagnosis?
   A. Mitral stenosis
   B. Mitral regurgitation
   C. Aortic stenosis
   D. Aortic regurgitation

3. What is the most common cause of papillary muscle rupture?
   A. Trauma
   B. Myocardial infarction
   C. Rheumatic heart disease
   D. Iatrogenic

4. What is the major valvular lesion in acute rheumatic fever?
   A. Mitral stenosis
   B. Mitral regurgitation
   C. Aortic stenosis
   D. Aortic regurgitation

Mitral Regurgitation

1. A and B

2. B

3. B

4. B

Reference

Walker CM, Reddy GP, Steiner RM: Radiology of the heart. Chapter 10. In Rosendorff C, editor: *Essential Cardiology*, ed 3, New York, 2013, Springer.

Cross-Reference

Cardiac Imaging: The REQUISITES, ed 3, pp 190-194.

Comment

Pathology and Etiology

Mitral regurgitation is caused by a malfunction of any part of the mitral apparatus, including the valve leaflets, chordae, papillary muscles, mitral annulus, and adjacent left ventricular wall. Causes of mitral regurgitation include ischemic cardiomyopathy, myocardial infarction, papillary muscle rupture, rheumatic heart disease, endocarditis, and trauma.

Imaging Findings and Diagnostic Criteria

Chest radiographic findings of mitral regurgitation vary depending on the chronicity and severity of disease. Acute severe mitral regurgitation results in pulmonary venous hypertension and alveolar edema without significant cardiac enlargement. After several days, the heart dilates, and interstitial edema persists. After weeks to months, the left atrium and ventricle are enlarged (Figs. A and B), and the pulmonary pattern is variable.

Echocardiography is commonly used to grade the severity of mitral regurgitation. MRI can be used to quantify the regurgitant fraction.

Notes

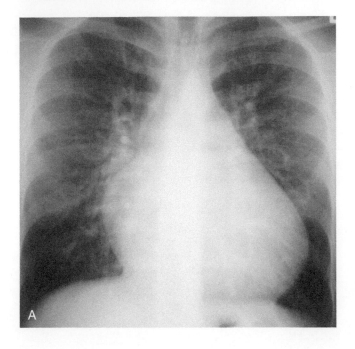

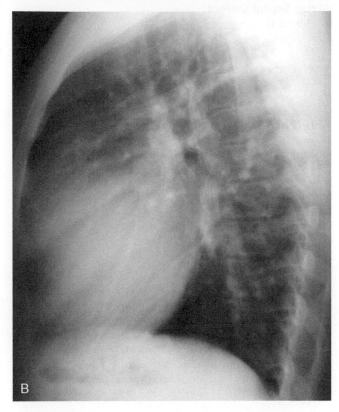

History: An acyanotic patient presents with a heart murmur.

1. What should be included in the differential diagnosis? (Choose all that apply.)
   A. Atrial septal defect (ASD)
   B. Ventricular septal defect (VSD)
   C. Patent ductus arteriosus (PDA)
   D. Partial anomalous pulmonary venous connection (PAPVC)

2. What is the most likely diagnosis?
   A. ASD
   B. VSD
   C. PDA
   D. PAPVC

3. What lesion is commonly associated with this anomaly?
   A. VSD
   B. PDA
   C. PAPVC
   D. Total anomalous pulmonary venous connection

4. Which anomaly can manifest with cyanosis and shunt vascularity on chest radiographs?
   A. Tetralogy of Fallot
   B. Ebstein anomaly
   C. Coarctation of the aorta
   D. Transposition of the great arteries

Atrial Septal Defect

1. A and D

2. A

3. C

4. D

Reference

Higgins CB: Radiography of congenital heart disease. In Webb WR, Higgins CB, editors: *Thoracic Imaging: Pulmonary and Cardiovascular Radiology*, ed 2, Philadelphia, 2010, Lippincott Williams & Wilkins.

Cross-Reference

Cardiac Imaging: The REQUISITES, ed 3, pp 335–338.

Comment

Types of Atrial Septal Defect

There are several types of ASD, including ostium secundum, ostium primum, and sinus venosus. Ostium secundum ASD is the most common type and is the most frequently diagnosed left-to-right shunt in adult patients. Ostium primum ASD is present in atrioventricular septal defect (formerly known as endocardial cushion defect). A sinus venosus defect is commonly associated with PAPVC.

Imaging Findings

Although the chest radiograph may be normal when the shunt is small, pulmonary vascularity is usually increased (shunt vascularity) (Figs. A and B). Typically, the main pulmonary artery, peripheral pulmonary branches, right atrium, and right ventricle are enlarged. The left atrium is not enlarged; this is an important sign that differentiates ASD from VSD or PDA. PAPVC is another atrial level shunt that can mimic ASD physiologically and can appear similar to ASD on a chest radiograph. Echocardiography can delineate the size and location of the ASD. MRI can be performed if echocardiography does not demonstrate a suspected ASD, and velocity-encoded cine phase contrast MRI can be used to quantify the severity of the shunt.

Notes

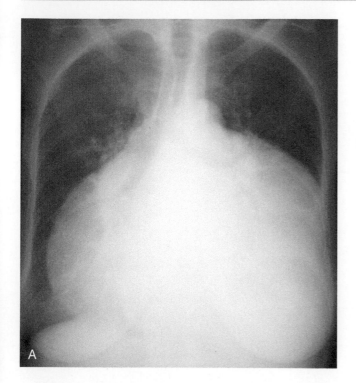

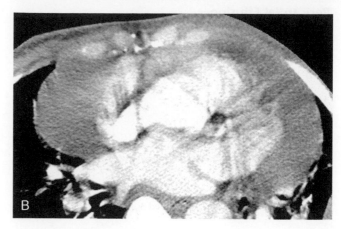

History: A patient presents with shortness of breath.

1. What should be included in the differential diagnosis for the appearance of the heart on the radiograph? (Choose all that apply.)
   A. Mitral stenosis
   B. Tricuspid regurgitation
   C. Dilated cardiomyopathy
   D. Pericardial effusion

2. What is the most likely diagnosis?
   A. Pericardial effusion
   B. Pericardial tumor
   C. Pericardial cyst
   D. Constrictive pericarditis

3. What finding is most specific for a malignant effusion?
   A. High-density fluid
   B. Nodularity
   C. Thickening
   D. Enhancement

4. What does pulsus paradoxus indicate?
   A. Tamponade
   B. Tumor
   C. Constriction
   D. Hemorrhage

Pericardial Effusion

1. B, C, and D

2. A

3. B

4. A

Reference

Yared K, Baggish AL, Picard MH, et al: Multimodality imaging of pericardial diseases, *JACC Cardiovasc Imaging* 3(6):650–660, 2010.

Cross-Reference

Cardiac Imaging: The REQUISITES, ed 3, pp 265–267.

Comment

Radiographic Features

A small pericardial effusion is frequently not identified on chest radiography. As the pericardial effusion increases, the cardiac silhouette may acquire a globular ("water bottle") configuration, which results from obscuration of the normal bulges and indentations of the cardiac contours (Fig. A). Because a pericardial effusion can cause enlargement of the cardiac silhouette, it may be difficult to distinguish pericardial effusion from cardiomegaly on chest radiographs. One differentiating feature is obscuration of the hilar vessels by a large pericardial effusion, which does not occur with cardiomegaly alone. Sometimes a pericardial effusion can cause an opaque band between the pericardial fat and the subpericardial fat on a lateral chest film, known as the "fat pad" sign. Although this sign is specific, its sensitivity for pericardial effusion is limited.

Cross-Sectional Imaging

Echocardiography is more sensitive than chest radiography for the diagnosis of pericardial effusion. When a pericardial effusion is suggested by clinical or radiographic findings, echocardiography can confirm the diagnosis. CT and MRI also can demonstrate pericardial effusion (Fig. B) and are useful for the identification of a hemorrhagic effusion and nodularity of the pericardium, both of which suggest a malignant effusion.

Notes

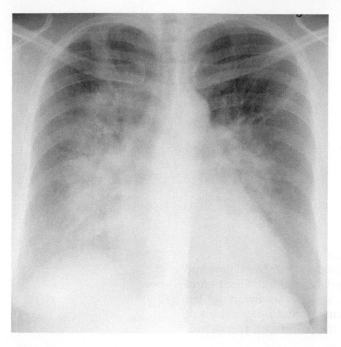

History: A patient presents with shortness of breath.

1. What should be included in the differential diagnosis? (Choose all that apply.)
   A. Fibrosis
   B. Pneumonia
   C. Pulmonary edema
   D. Acute respiratory distress syndrome

2. What is the predominant distribution of the lung opacity?
   A. Basilar
   B. Upper lobe
   C. Peripheral
   D. Perihilar

3. What is the most likely diagnosis?
   A. Fibrosis
   B. Pneumonia
   C. Pulmonary edema
   D. Acute respiratory distress syndrome

4. What is the most likely etiology?
   A. Cardiogenic
   B. Neurogenic
   C. Fluid overload
   D. Congenital heart disease

Pulmonary Edema

1. B, C, and D

2. D

3. C

4. A

Reference

Eisenhuber E, Schaefer-Prokop CM, Prosch H, et al: Bedside chest radiography, *Respir Care* 57(3):427–443, 2012.

Cross-Reference

Cardiac Imaging: The REQUISITES, ed 3, p 18.

Comment

Pathophysiology and Etiology

Pulmonary edema can be related to both blood flow and blood pressure or to blood pressure alone. Elevation of pulmonary venous pressure can be secondary to left ventricular failure, mitral stenosis, and other causes of vascular obstruction distal to the pulmonary arterial bed.

Imaging Findings

When pressure increases, pulmonary blood flow is redistributed to the upper lobes, which manifests as enlargement of the upper lobe vessels ("cephalization") on chest radiographs. When pulmonary venous pressure increases further, pulmonary interstitial edema ensues. Kerley B lines—thin, horizontal, interlobular septal lines—are seen at the lung bases on chest radiographs. With further elevation of pulmonary venous pressure, alveolar edema develops, and chest radiographs may demonstrate opacities that involve the central portions of the lungs, sometimes producing a "bat wing" appearance (Figure). If the pulmonary edema is related to congestive heart failure, the cardiac silhouette is enlarged, and pleural effusions are often seen on chest radiographs.

Notes

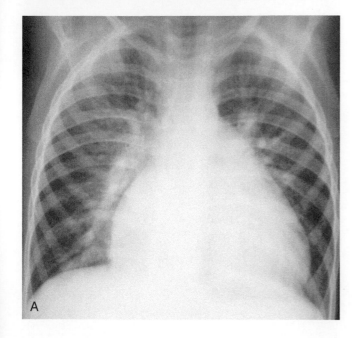

A

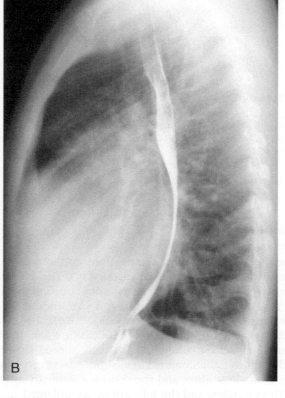

B

History: An acyanotic patient presents with a heart murmur.

1. What should be included in the differential diagnosis? (Choose all that apply.)
   A. Atrial septal defect (ASD)
   B. Ventricular septal defect (VSD)
   C. Patent ductus arteriosus (PDA)
   D. Partial anomalous pulmonary venous connection (PAPVC)

2. What is the most likely diagnosis?
   A. ASD
   B. VSD
   C. PDA
   D. PAPVC

3. What lesion commonly causes enlargement of the left atrium?
   A. VSD
   B. ASD
   C. PAPVC
   D. Total anomalous pulmonary venous connection (TAPVC)

4. Which anomaly can manifest with cyanosis and shunt vascularity on chest radiographs?
   A. Tetralogy of Fallot
   B. PAPVC
   C. Pulmonary stenosis
   D. TAPVC

Ventricular Septal Defect

1. B and C

2. B

3. A

4. D

Reference

Higgins CB: Radiography of congenital heart disease. In Webb WR, Higgins CB, editors: *Thoracic Imaging: Pulmonary and Cardiovascular Radiology*, ed 2, Philadelphia, 2010, Lippincott Williams & Wilkins.

Cross-Reference

Cardiac Imaging: The REQUISITES, ed 3, pp 340–342.

Comment

Radiography

The chest radiographs demonstrate cardiomegaly and shunt vascularity (increased vascularity). The left atrium is enlarged, signifying that the shunt is beyond the atrial level. The aortic knob is normal in size, indicating that the most likely lesion in an acyanotic patient is a VSD. PDA typically causes dilation of the aortic knob. If a VSD is small, the chest radiograph is usually normal. However, if the left-to-right shunt is large, shunt vascularity is identified on chest films, and the central pulmonary arteries, both ventricles, and the left atrium are enlarged.

Cross-Sectional Imaging

Echocardiography usually demonstrates the location and size of the defect. MRI may be performed in certain patients to evaluate associated abnormalities or to define certain lesions such as a supracristal VSD, which may be difficult to image by echocardiography. Velocity-encoded cine phase contrast MRI can be performed to quantify the pulmonary-to-systemic flow ratio, which is an indicator of the severity of the shunt.

Notes

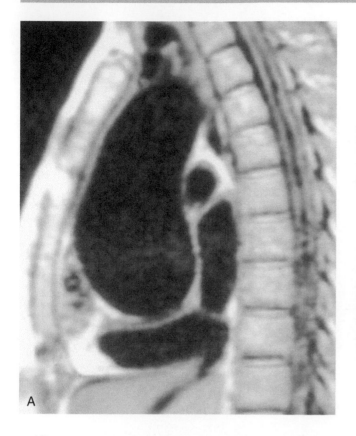

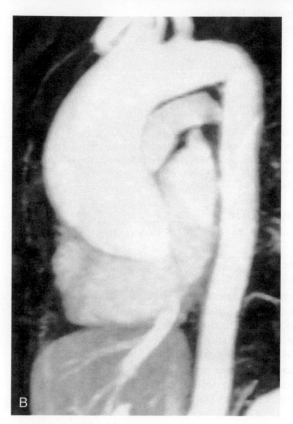

History: A patient presents with a lanky body habitus.

1. What are etiologies for this appearance? (Choose all that apply.)
   A. Ehlers-Danlos syndrome
   B. Marfan syndrome
   C. Atherosclerosis
   D. Syphilis

2. What is the most likely diagnosis?
   A. Ehlers-Danlos syndrome
   B. Marfan syndrome
   C. Atherosclerosis
   D. Syphilis

3. Which of the following is not a complication of this condition?
   A. Rupture
   B. Penetrating ulcer
   C. Dissection
   D. Aortic regurgitation

4. Which MRI technique could be used to quantify aortic regurgitation?
   A. Double inversion recovery (black blood)
   B. Late gadolinium enhancement
   C. Phase contrast
   D. Magnetic resonance angiography (MRA)

Annuloaortic Ectasia

1. A and B

2. B

3. B

4. C

Reference

Reddy GP, Gunn M, Mitsumori LM, et al: Multislice CT and MRI of the thoracic aorta. In Webb WR, Higgins CB, editors: *Thoracic Imaging: Pulmonary and Cardiovascular Radiology*, ed 2, Philadelphia, 2010, Lippincott Williams & Wilkins.

Cross-Reference

Cardiac Imaging: The REQUISITES, ed 3, pp 388–389.

Comment

Pathology and Etiology

Enlargement of the aortic root and ascending aorta is characteristic of annuloaortic ectasia. The dilation of the aorta in this condition may stop at the sinotubular junction or extend to involve the entire ascending aorta, which is sometimes called the "tulip bulb" configuration. Annuloaortic ectasia results from cystic medial necrosis, which can be idiopathic or can be associated with Marfan syndrome or Ehlers-Danlos syndrome.

Complications

Complications of annuloaortic ectasia include aortic dissection, aortic rupture, and aortic regurgitation. Although 5.5–6 cm is the usual threshold of aortic diameter that necessitates surgery, operative repair may be indicated in annuloaortic ectasia when the aorta reaches a diameter of 5 cm owing to the high risk of rupture.

Imaging

MRI and CT are the most appropriate modalities for imaging of annuloaortic ectasia. MRI has the advantages of no ionizing radiation and the capability to provide quantitative assessment of aortic regurgitation (Figs. A and B).

Notes

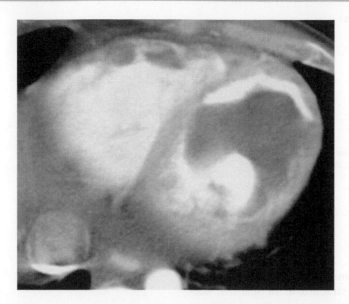

History: A patient presents with a hematologic disorder.

1. Which cardiac chambers are abnormal? (Choose all that apply.)
   A. Left atrium
   B. Left ventricle
   C. Right atrium
   D. Right ventricle

2. What is the most common mass in the heart?
   A. Thrombus
   B. Myxoma
   C. Metastasis
   D. Angiosarcoma

3. What is the most likely diagnosis?
   A. Thrombus
   B. Myxoma
   C. Metastasis
   D. Angiosarcoma

4. Which imaging modality is most specific for differentiating a thrombus from a neoplasm?
   A. Echocardiography
   B. CT
   C. MRI
   D. Angiography

Left Ventricular Thrombus

1. B and D

2. A

3. A

4. C

Reference

Tatli S, Lipton MJ: CT for intracardiac thrombi and tumors, *Int J Cardiovasc Imaging* 21(1):115-131, 2005.

Cross-Reference

Cardiac Imaging: The REQUISITES, ed 3, p 274.

Comment

Cardiac Masses

Thrombus is the most common cardiac or paracardiac mass. Among cardiac and paracardiac neoplasms, secondary tumors occur at 40 times the rate of primary neoplasms. Secondary tumors can involve the heart by direct extension (most commonly lymphoma or lymphadenopathy metastatic from lung or breast carcinoma) or by hematogenous spread (most commonly lung or breast carcinoma or melanoma). Primary benign tumors of the heart include myxoma, lipoma, and rhabdomyoma (associated with tuberous sclerosis). Primary malignant neoplasms include angiosarcoma and rhabdomyosarcoma.

Imaging Findings and Diagnostic Criteria

Echocardiography and CT can identify cardiac masses (Figure). MRI is the most accurate imaging examination for differentiating tumor from thrombus. Neoplasms enhance homogeneously or heterogeneously after administration of gadolinium-chelate contrast agent, whereas bland thrombi typically do not enhance except in the periphery. On steady-state free precession (SSFP) MRI, a tumor usually shows intermediate signal intensity, and thrombus tends to show low signal intensity. However, myxomas can contain calcium, and iron-containing areas can be dark on SSFP images.

Notes

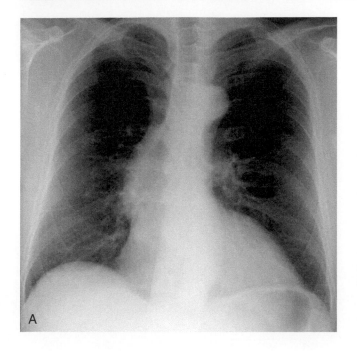

A

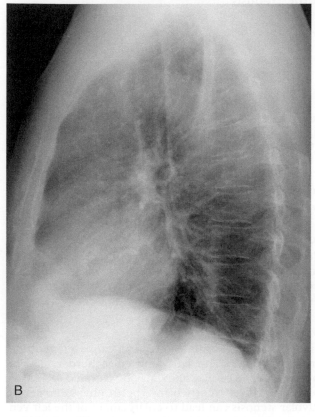

B

History: A patient presents with easy fatigability.

1. What should be included in the differential diagnosis? (Choose all that apply.)
   A. Coarctation of the aorta
   B. Systemic hypertension
   C. Aortic stenosis
   D. Syphilis

2. What is the most likely diagnosis?
   A. Coarctation of the aorta
   B. Systemic hypertension
   C. Aortic stenosis
   D. Syphilis

3. Which MRI technique could be used to quantify aortic stenosis?
   A. Double inversion recovery (black blood)
   B. Delayed enhancement
   C. Phase contrast
   D. Magnetic resonance angiography (MRA)

4. If the peak velocity across the valve is 3 m/s, what is the pressure gradient?
   A. 3 mm Hg
   B. 9 mm Hg
   C. 12 m Hg
   D. 36 mm Hg

Aortic Stenosis

1. B and C

2. C

3. C

4. D

Reference

Walker CM, Reddy GP, Steiner RM: Radiology of the heart. Chapter 10. In Rosendorff C, editor: *Essential Cardiology*, ed 3, New York, 2013, Springer.

Cross-Reference

Cardiac Imaging: The REQUISITES, ed 3, pp 172–177.

Comment

Etiology

Isolated stenosis of the aortic valve is most commonly secondary to congenital bicuspid valve. Rheumatic heart disease is another important cause of aortic stenosis.

Imaging Features

Mild-to-moderate aortic stenosis can cause left ventricular hypertrophy. The left ventricular border may be rounded, or the cardiac apex may be elevated secondary to concentric left ventricular hypertrophy. More severe valvular stenosis can lead to enlargement of the left ventricle and atrium and to hypertrophy. The ascending aortic contour bulges rightward secondary to poststenotic dilation (Fig. A). Calcification of the valve can develop as a result of degeneration and can be seen on CT or, when severe, on chest radiographs (Fig. B).

Quantification

The pressure gradient across the valve can be calculated by use of the modified Bernoulli equation: $\Delta P = 4v^2$, where *P* is the pressure in mm Hg and *v* is peak velocity in m/s. The peak velocity can be estimated by echocardiography or velocity-encoded cine phase contrast MRI.

Notes

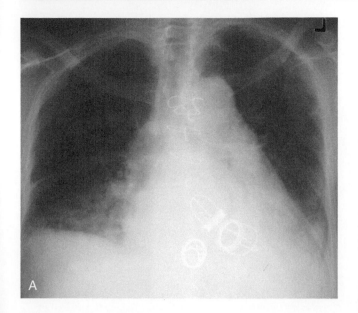

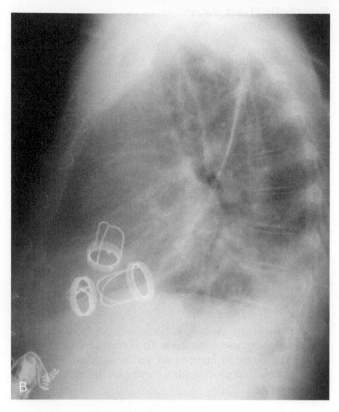

History: A patient presents with shortness of breath.

1. Which valves have been replaced? (Choose all that apply.)
   A. Aortic
   B. Mitral
   C. Pulmonary
   D. Tricuspid

2. What is the most common cause of multivalve disease?
   A. Congenital valve disease
   B. Carcinoid syndrome
   C. Marfan syndrome
   D. Rheumatic heart disease

3. What is the primary advantage of a tissue valve prosthesis over a mechanical valve prosthesis?
   A. Safer in the MRI environment
   B. No need for anticoagulation
   C. Greater durability of valve
   D. Less likelihood of calcification

4. Which MRI technique could be used to quantify regurgitation of a prosthetic valve?
   A. Double inversion recovery (black blood)
   B. Delayed enhancement
   C. Phase contrast
   D. Magnetic resonance angiography (MRA)

Prosthetic Heart Valves

1. A, B, and D

2. D

3. B

4. C

References

Steiner RM, Mintz G, Morse D, et al: The radiology of cardiac valve prostheses, *Radiographics* 8(2):277-298, 1988.

Walker CM, Reddy GP, Steiner RM: Radiology of the heart. In Rosendorff C, editor: *Essential Cardiology*, ed 3, New York, 2013, Springer.

MRIsafety.com. http://www.mrisafety.com/. Accessed February 14, 2013.

Cross-Reference

Cardiac Imaging: The REQUISITES, ed 3, pp 49-50.

Comment

Etiology and Treatment

Rheumatic heart disease is the most common cause of three-valve disease. Patients with three-valve disease may present with heart failure and severe cardiomegaly. Surgical correction is complex, and the mortality rate is approximately 5%.

Types of Prosthetic Valves

Typically, prosthetic mitral and aortic valves are mechanical, and a tricuspid prosthesis may be mechanical or a tissue valve (bioprosthesis). A bioprosthesis can be a heterograft (porcine), a homograft (from a cadaver), or an autograft, in which the patient's own pulmonary valve and root are used to replace the aortic valve and root. When an autograft is used, a homograft is placed into the pulmonary position.

Imaging Features

Mechanical prostheses have various radiographic appearances, and some are radiolucent (Figs. A and B). Patients who have a mechanical prosthesis require anticoagulation. Typically, bioprostheses have a single radiopaque ring.

Notes

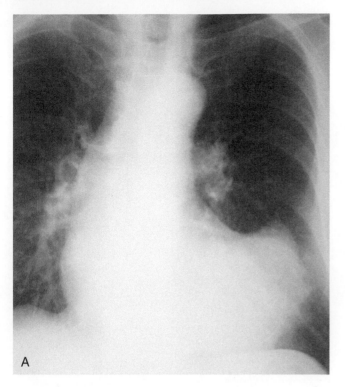

A

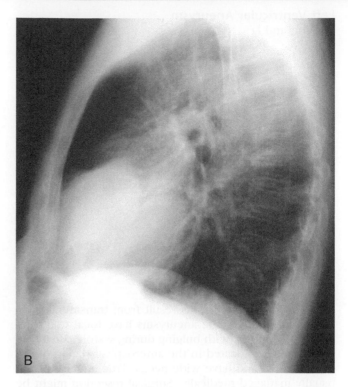

B

History: A patient presents with chest pain.

1. What should be included in the differential diagnosis? (Choose all that apply.)
   A. Mitral regurgitation
   B. Ventricular aneurysm
   C. Pericardial tumor
   D. Pericardial cyst

2. What is the most likely diagnosis?
   A. Mitral regurgitation
   B. Ventricular aneurysm
   C. Pericardial tumor
   D. Pericardial cyst

3. What is the most common cause of left ventricular aneurysm?
   A. Trauma
   B. Iatrogenic injury
   C. Myocardial infarction
   D. Tumor

4. On CT or MRI, what is the most reliable feature to distinguish a true aneurysm from a false aneurysm?
   A. Size of ostium
   B. Size of aneurysm
   C. Location
   D. Wall thickness

CASE 35

Left Ventricular Aneurysm

1. B, C, and D

2. B

3. C

4. A

References

Walker CM, Reddy GP, Steiner RM: Radiology of the heart. In Rosendorff C, editor: *Essential Cardiology*, ed 3, New York, 2013, Springer.

White RD: MR and CT assessment for ischemic cardiac disease, *J Magn Reson Imaging* 19(6):659–675, 2004.

Cross-Reference

Cardiac Imaging: The REQUISITES, ed 3, pp 235–237.

Comment

Pathology and Etiology

Left ventricular aneurysms result from transmural myocardial infarction. True aneurysms have focal wall thinning and akinesis, with bulging during systole. Most true aneurysms are located in the anteroapical region of the left ventricle and have wide necks. True aneurysms are usually managed medically. Surgical resection might be needed in the setting of poor ventricular function. A false aneurysm is actually a contained rupture. Most false aneurysms are inferoposterior in location and are connected to the left ventricle via a narrow neck. False aneurysms are usually treated surgically.

Imaging Findings and Diagnostic Criteria

Radiographs may show a contour abnormality along the left ventricle (Figs. A and B). Calcification may be present. With MRI or CT, true and false aneurysms can be differentiated on the basis of their ostia. A true aneurysm typically has an ostium that is greater than 50% of the aneurysm diameter, whereas a false aneurysm typically has an ostium that is less than 50% of the aneurysm diameter.

Notes

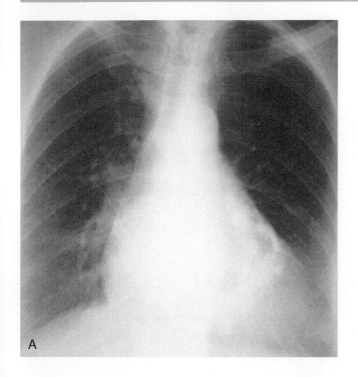

A

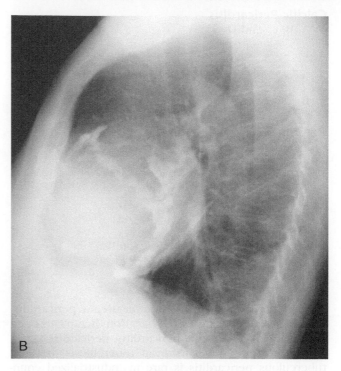

B

History: A patient presents with dyspnea on exertion and lower extremity edema.

1. What etiologies can cause this finding? (Choose all that apply.)
   A. Uremia
   B. Hemorrhage
   C. Viral infection
   D. Tuberculosis

2. Which structure is calcified?
   A. Coronary artery
   B. Left ventricle
   C. Valve
   D. Pericardium

3. Given the symptoms, what is the most likely diagnosis?
   A. Acute pericarditis
   B. Constrictive pericarditis
   C. Tamponade
   D. Tumor

4. What is the most appropriate treatment?
   A. Antibiotics
   B. Pericardial stripping
   C. Pericardiocentesis
   D. Radiation therapy

Calcific Pericarditis

1. A, B, C, and D

2. D

3. B

4. B

References

Gowda RM, Boxt LM: Calcifications of the heart, *Radiol Clin North Am* 42(3):603-617, vi-vii, 2004.

Walker CM, Reddy GP, Steiner RM: Radiology of the heart. In Rosendorff C, editor: *Essential Cardiology*, ed 3, New York, 2013, Springer.

Cross-Reference

Cardiac Imaging: The REQUISITES, ed 3, pp 10, 79-82.

Comment

Calcific Pericarditis

Chronic pericarditis can occur after uremic pericarditis, viral or tuberculous infection, radiation therapy, or open heart surgery. In chronic pericarditis, pericardial calcification most often results from tuberculosis. Because tuberculous pericarditis is rare in industrialized countries, pericardial calcification (Figs. A and B) occurs in less than 20% of patients with chronic pericarditis. Calcific pericarditis does not cause symptoms of constriction.

Constrictive Pericarditis

In the setting of chronic pericarditis, a patient may have constrictive pericarditis. Constrictive pericarditis is difficult to distinguish from restrictive cardiomyopathy. If a patient has constrictive or restrictive physiology, characterized by dyspnea, lower extremity edema, pleural effusions, and ascites, imaging studies can be used to differentiate constrictive pericarditis from restrictive cardiomyopathy. Pericardial thickening of at least 4 mm (best seen on MRI or CT), pericardial calcification (Figs. A and B), or abnormal diastolic septal motion ("bounce") establishes the diagnosis of constrictive pericarditis.

Notes

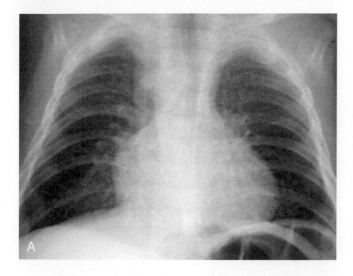

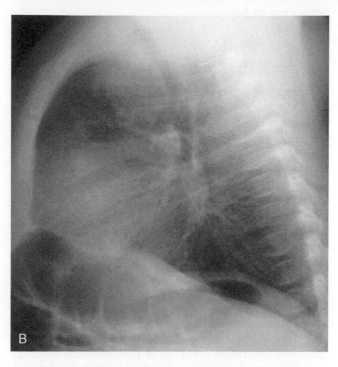

History: A child presents with cyanosis.

1. What should be included in the differential diagnosis? (Choose all that apply.)
   A. Ebstein anomaly
   B. Truncus arteriosus
   C. Tetralogy of Fallot
   D. Pulmonary atresia with ventricular septal defect

2. What is the most likely diagnosis?
   A. Ebstein anomaly
   B. Truncus arteriosus
   C. Tetralogy of Fallot
   D. Pulmonary atresia with ventricular septal defect

3. Tetralogy of Fallot comprises all of the following *except:*
   A. Right aortic arch
   B. Overriding aorta
   C. Pulmonary infundibular stenosis
   D. Ventricular septal defect
   E. Right ventricular hypertrophy

4. Which of the following is a severe variant of tetralogy of Fallot?
   A. Truncus arteriosus
   B. Pulmonary atresia with ventricular septal defect
   C. Ebstein anomaly
   D. Transposition of the great arteries

Tetralogy of Fallot

1. C and D

2. C

3. A

4. B

Reference

Higgins CB: Radiography of congenital heart disease. In Webb WR, Higgins CB, editors: *Thoracic Imaging: Pulmonary and Cardiovascular Radiology*, ed 2, Philadelphia, 2010, Lippincott Williams & Wilkins, pp 742-767.

Cross-Reference

Cardiac Imaging: The REQUISITES, ed 3, pp 359-367.

Comment

Tetralogy of Fallot Overview

Tetralogy of Fallot is the most common cyanotic congenital heart disease in children and adults. The lesions of tetralogy of Fallot are ventricular septal defect, pulmonary infundibular stenosis, right ventricular hypertrophy, and overriding aorta. Most patients with tetralogy of Fallot have decreased pulmonary vascularity, but vascularity can be normal if the infundibular stenosis is mild. Approximately 25% of patients have a right aortic arch. Pulmonary stenosis can occur at multiple levels, including subvalvular or infundibular (most common), valvular, supravalvular, and peripheral.

Pulmonary Atresia with Ventricular Septal Defect

Pulmonary atresia with ventricular septal defect is a severe variant of tetralogy of Fallot in which the pulmonary valve is atretic. Blood reaches the lungs via systemic-to-pulmonary collateral vessels.

Imaging

In tetralogy of Fallot, radiographs typically demonstrate decreased vascularity, concavity of the pulmonary artery segment, and sometimes an upturned cardiac apex. Chest radiograph in an infant typically demonstrates normal to decreased pulmonary vascularity, normal heart size, and a right aortic arch (Figs. A and B). Echocardiography and angiography are usually performed preoperatively. MRI and CT are occasionally performed preoperatively. MRI is often performed after surgical repair to monitor right ventricular function and to identify and quantify pulmonary regurgitation, which is a complication of surgery.

Notes

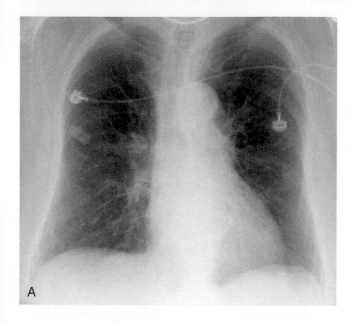

A

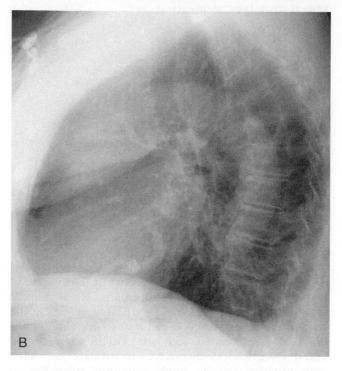

B

History: A patient presents with chest pain.

1. Which letters of the alphabet can be used to describe the configuration of the calcification? (Choose all that apply.)
   A. C
   B. J
   C. L
   D. S
   E. O

2. Which structure is calcified?
   A. Aortic valve
   B. Aortic annulus
   C. Mitral valve
   D. Mitral annulus

3. What is the most common cause of this finding?
   A. Rheumatic heart disease
   B. Endocarditis
   C. Degenerative
   D. Congenital bicuspid valve

4. What valvular lesion is most commonly associated with this finding?
   A. Mitral stenosis
   B. Mitral regurgitation
   C. Aortic stenosis
   D. Aortic regurgitation

Mitral Annular Calcification

1. A, B, and E

2. D

3. C

4. B

Reference

Gowda RM, Boxt LM: Calcifications of the heart, *Radiol Clin North Am* 42(3):603-617, vi, vii, 2004.

Cross-Reference

Cardiac Imaging: The REQUISITES, ed 3, pp 8-9.

Comment

Pathology and Etiology

Mitral annular calcification is typically degenerative and related to aging. It occurs more frequently in women and in patients with chronic renal failure. Mitral annular calcification rarely causes symptoms, but when the calcification is extensive, it can lead to mitral regurgitation (or rarely mitral stenosis). Calcification of the mitral valve leaflets themselves is strongly associated with valvular stenosis, most commonly secondary to rheumatic disease.

Imaging Findings and Diagnostic Criteria

Radiographs show calcification of the mitral annulus in a "J," reverse "C," or "O" shape (Figs. A and B). It is important to differentiate mitral annular calcification from other calcified cardiac structures on chest radiography. Aortic valve calcification is more anterior than mitral annular calcification and when seen on chest radiography usually indicates at least moderate or severe valvular stenosis. Pericardial calcification is often localized to the atrioventricular groove or can circumferentially surround the heart. It is associated with tuberculosis pericarditis, uremic pericarditis, and radiation therapy and may indicate constrictive pericarditis in the appropriate clinical context. Rarely, intracardiac tumors such as myxoma can calcify diffusely or peripherally.

Notes

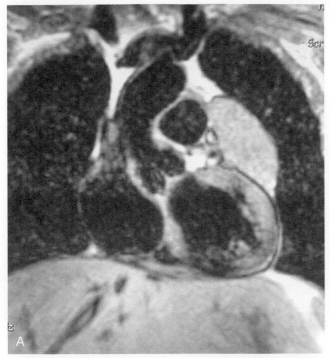

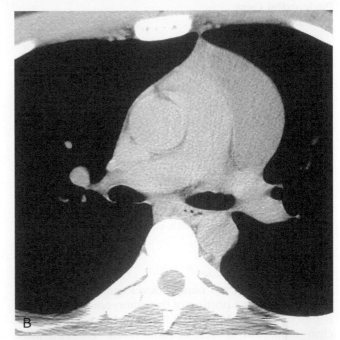

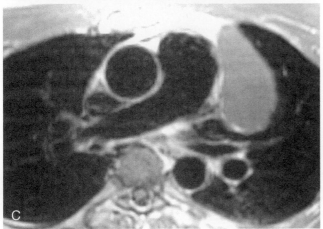

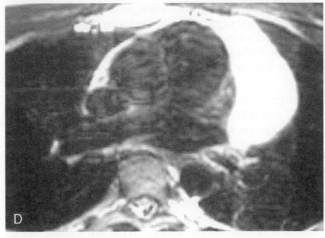

History: A patient has a mediastinal abnormality on chest radiography.

1. What etiologies can cause this finding? (Choose all that apply.)
   A. Thymoma
   B. Thymic cyst
   C. Pericardial cyst
   D. Lymphoma

2. What is the most likely diagnosis?
   A. Thymoma
   B. Thymic cyst
   C. Pericardial cyst
   D. Lymphoma

3. What is the most common location of a pericardial cyst?
   A. Right cardiophrenic sulcus
   B. Left cardiophrenic sulcus
   C. Superior pericardial recess
   D. Subcarinal

4. Which of the following is least specific for a pericardial cyst?
   A. Hounsfield number of 10 on non–contrast-enhanced CT scan
   B. Hounsfield number of 30 on both non–contrast-enhanced CT scan and contrast-enhanced CT scan
   C. Low signal intensity on T1-weighted MRI
   D. High signal intensity on T2-weighted MRI

Pericardial Cyst

1. B and C

2. C

3. A

4. B

References

Kim JS, Kim HH, Yoon Y: Imaging of pericardial diseases, *Clin Radiol* 62(7):626–631, 2007.

Wang ZJ, Reddy GP, Gotway MB, et al: CT and MR imaging of pericardial disease, *Radiographics* 23(Spec No):S167–S180, 2003.

Cross-Reference

Cardiac Imaging: The REQUISITES, ed 3, pp 78–79.

Comment

Etiology and Pathology

A pericardial cyst is a benign developmental lesion that is formed when a portion of the embryonic pericardium is pinched off and isolated. It has a thin wall, contains clear fluid, and is well circumscribed. The two most common locations are the right and left cardiophrenic angles. When a pericardial cyst is located in another area of the mediastinum, it can be difficult to differentiate from a bronchogenic, esophageal duplication, neuroenteric, or thymic cyst.

Imaging Features and Diagnosis

On CT and MRI, pericardial cysts are round or ovoid and are contiguous with the normal pericardium (Fig. A). CT scan shows a well-circumscribed mass (Fig. B). The density may be in the range of simple fluid, in which case the diagnosis is straightforward. If the density is higher, non–contrast-enhanced and contrast-enhanced CT scans can be performed to assess for enhancement. Pericardial cysts do not enhance, in contrast to neoplasms. On MRI, these lesions typically exhibit signal characteristics consistent with simple cysts found elsewhere in the body. The lesions manifest as low to intermediate signal masses on T1-weighted images (Fig. C) and high signal intensity lesions on T2-weighted images (Fig. D).

Notes

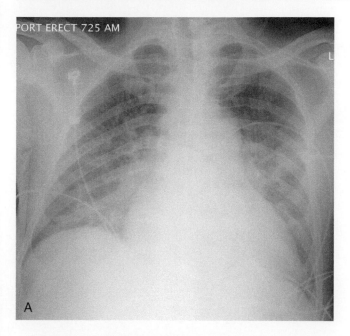

A

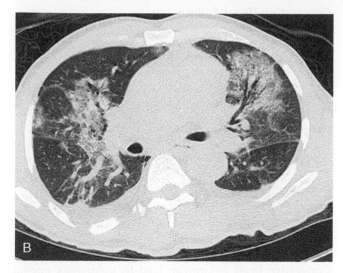

B

History: A patient presents with shortness of breath.

1. What should be included in the differential diagnosis? (Choose all that apply.)
   A. Viral pneumonia
   B. Cryptogenic organizing pneumonia
   C. Pulmonary edema
   D. Acute respiratory distress syndrome

2. What is the predominant distribution of the lung opacity?
   A. Basilar
   B. Upper lobe
   C. Peripheral
   D. Diffuse and uniform

3. What is the most likely diagnosis?
   A. Bacterial pneumonia
   B. Cryptogenic organizing pneumonia
   C. Pulmonary edema
   D. Acute respiratory distress syndrome

4. What is the most likely etiology?
   A. Cardiogenic
   B. Neurogenic
   C. Fluid overload
   D. Congenital heart disease

Congestive Heart Failure

1. A, C, and D

2. A

3. C

4. A

Reference

Eisenhuber E, Schaefer-Prokop CM, Prosch H, et al: Bedside chest radiography, *Respir Care* 57(3):427–443, 2012.

Cross-Reference

Cardiac Imaging: The REQUISITES, ed 3, p 18.

Comment

Pathophysiology and Etiology

Congestive heart failure can lead to pulmonary edema and pleural effusions. Pulmonary edema is related to both blood flow and blood pressure or to blood pressure alone. Elevation of pulmonary venous pressure can be secondary to left ventricular failure, mitral stenosis, and other causes of vascular obstruction distal to the pulmonary arterial bed.

Imaging Findings

Patients with congestive heart failure typically have pulmonary edema, as evidenced by diffuse lung disease (Fig. A) or Kerley B lines on radiography. Early signs of pulmonary edema include subpleural thickening, best visualized along pulmonary fissures, and indistinct vessel margins. CT scan can show ground-glass opacity (Fig. B), interlobular septal thickening, and frank consolidation. The lung opacity is often perihilar or basilar predominant (or both). In patients with alveolar edema, there may be central opacities with sparing of the lung periphery—so-called bat-wing pulmonary edema. If the pulmonary edema is related to congestive heart failure, the cardiac silhouette is enlarged, and pleural effusions are often seen on chest radiography. The radiographic findings of pulmonary edema often persist for hours to days after symptom resolution.

Cephalization

Acute pulmonary edema rarely causes redistribution of blood flow to the lung apices—so-called cephalization. Cephalization is usually seen in patients with long-standing pulmonary venous hypertension and occurs most commonly in patients with chronic mitral stenosis or long-standing left heart failure.

Notes

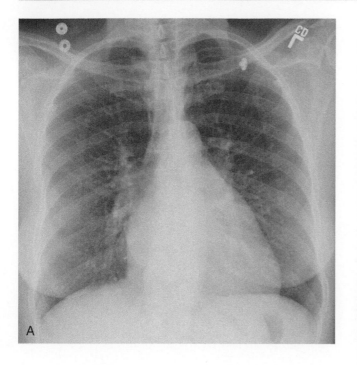

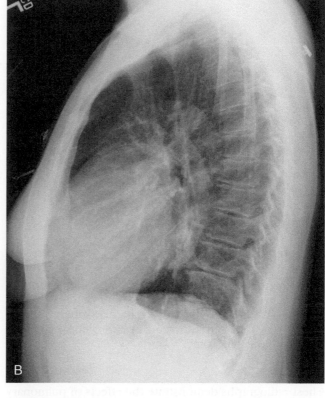

History: A patient presents with fatigue.

1. Which cardiac chambers are enlarged? (Choose all that apply.)
   A. Left atrium
   B. Left ventricle
   C. Right atrium
   D. Right ventricle

2. What is the most likely diagnosis?
   A. Mitral stenosis
   B. Mitral regurgitation
   C. Aortic stenosis
   D. Aortic regurgitation

3. What is the most common cause of mitral stenosis?
   A. Trauma
   B. Congenital
   C. Rheumatic heart disease
   D. Carcinoid syndrome

4. Which of the following lesions most commonly mimics the symptoms of mitral stenosis?
   A. Lipoma
   B. Myxoma
   C. Rhabdomyoma
   D. Fibroma

Mitral Stenosis

1. A

2. A

3. C

4. B

References

Bonow RO, Cheitlin MD, Crawford MH, et al: Task Force 3: valvular heart disease, *J Am Coll Cardiol* 45(8):1334–1340, 2005.

Walker CM, Reddy GP, Steiner RM: Radiology of the heart. In Rosendorff C, editor: *Essential Cardiology*, ed 3, Philadelphia, 2012, Saunders.

Cross-Reference

Cardiac Imaging: The REQUISITES, ed 3, pp 186–191.

Comment

Etiology

Mitral stenosis is usually acquired and develops approximately 5 to 10 years after an episode of rheumatic heart disease. Other causes of left atrial enlargement include prolapse of a left atrial myxoma or thrombus, amyloid, and carcinoid syndrome.

Radiography

Chest radiographs demonstrate the effects of pulmonary venous hypertension. The left atrium is enlarged, and the left ventricle is normal in size (Figs. A and B). Disproportionate enlargement of the left atrial appendage is often seen in rheumatic mitral stenosis. The mitral valve may contain nodular, amorphous calcification. Pulmonary interstitial edema is a frequent finding. Uncommonly, patients develop hemosiderosis and ossification of pulmonary nodules.

Cross-Sectional Imaging

Further evaluation involves echocardiography. The area of the valve is measured, and valve mobility, thickening of the leaflets, and submitral scarring are assessed. Velocity-encoded cine phase contrast MRI can be performed to quantify the severity of stenosis. The pressure gradient across the valve can be calculated by use of the modified Bernoulli equation, $\Delta P = 4v^2$, where P is the pressure in mm Hg and v is peak velocity in m/sec. The peak velocity can be estimated by echocardiography or by velocity-encoded cine phase contrast MRI.

Notes

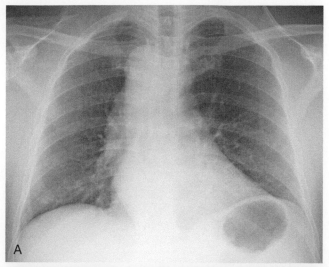

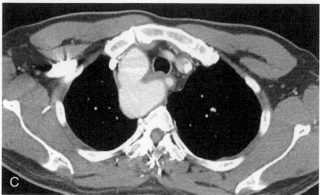

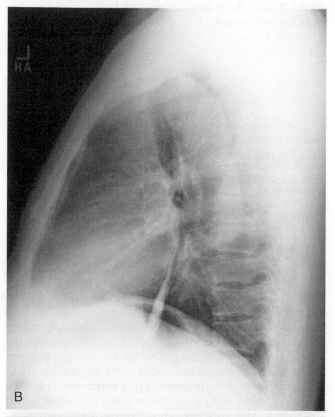

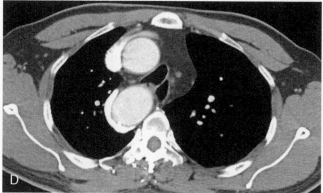

History: A patient presents with wheezing.

1. What should be included in the differential diagnosis based on the posteroanterior radiograph? (Choose all that apply.)
   A. Cervical aortic arch
   B. Double aortic arch
   C. Right aortic arch with aberrant left subclavian artery
   D. Mirror-image right aortic arch

2. Based on the posteroanterior and lateral radiographs, what is the most likely diagnosis?
   A. Cervical aortic arch
   B. Double aortic arch
   C. Right aortic arch with aberrant left subclavian artery
   D. Mirror-image right aortic arch

3. What is the clinical significance of this anomaly?
   A. Most patients have cyanotic congenital heart disease.
   B. It is associated with coarctation of the aorta.
   C. It causes subclavian steal syndrome.
   D. It is a vascular ring.

4. In this anomaly, what completes the ring on the left side?
   A. Left subclavian artery
   B. Left common carotid artery
   C. Ligamentum arteriosum and pulmonary artery
   D. Left aortic arch

CASE 42

Right Aortic Arch with Aberrant Left Subclavian Artery

1. C and D

2. C

3. D

4. C

References

Reddy GP, Higgins CB: Magnetic resonance imaging of congenital heart disease: evaluation of morphology and function, *Semin Roentgenol* 38(4):342-351, 2003.

Stojanovska J, Cascade PN, Chong S, et al: Embryology and imaging review of aortic arch anomalies, *J Thorac Imaging* 27(2):73-84, 2012.

Cross-Reference

Cardiac Imaging: The REQUISITES, ed 3, pp 413-414.

Comment

Clinical Features

A right aortic arch with an aberrant left subclavian artery is a congenital vascular ring (Figs. A-D). The ring is completed by the left-sided ligamentum arteriosum. Because there is a ring around the trachea and esophagus, these two structures are compressed to a variable extent. The most common symptoms are wheezing, dyspnea, and dysphagia, and patients often exhibit these symptoms during early childhood. The retroesophageal aberrant left subclavian artery may originate from a dilation, known as a diverticulum of Kommerell (Fig. C), which tends to exacerbate the compression on the trachea and esophagus. This type of right aortic arch is weakly associated (5% to 10%) with congenital heart disease, in contrast to the strong association of a mirror-image right arch (>95%).

Imaging and Diagnosis

MRI and CT can depict the vascular anatomy and the compression of the trachea and esophagus (Figs. C-D). Cine MRI has the added advantage of demonstrating dynamic compression of the trachea during pulsation of the aorta and arch vessels.

Notes

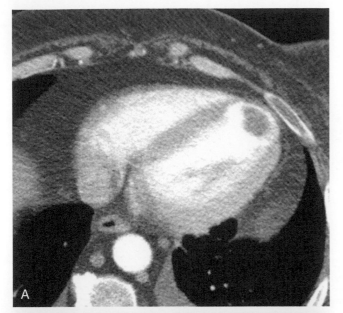

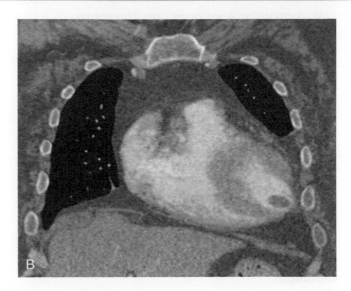

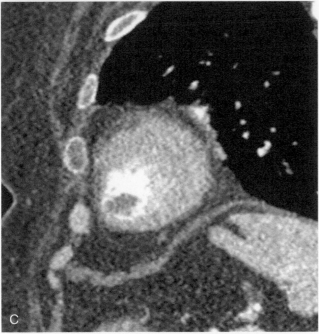

History: A patient presents with a history of myocardial infarction.

1. Which cardiac chambers are abnormal? (Choose all that apply.)
   A. Left atrium
   B. Left ventricle
   C. Right atrium
   D. Right ventricle

2. What is the most likely diagnosis?
   A. Thrombus
   B. Myxoma
   C. Metastasis
   D. Angiosarcoma

3. What is the most likely etiology of the abnormality?
   A. Arrhythmia
   B. Aortic stenosis
   C. Aneurysm
   D. Coagulation disorder

4. What is the most appropriate way to establish the diagnosis?
   A. Echocardiography
   B. MRI
   C. Angiography
   D. Biopsy

Left Ventricular Aneurysm and Thrombus

1. B

2. A

3. C

4. B

References

Chung JH, Mitsumori LM, Ordovas KG, et al: Heart as a source of stroke: imaging evaluation with computed tomography, *J Thorac Imaging* 27(3):W52–W60, 2012.⊙

Tatli S, Lipton MJ: CT for intracardiac thrombi and tumors, *Int J Cardiovasc Imaging* 21(1):115–131, 2005.⊙

Cross-Reference

Cardiac Imaging: The REQUISITES, ed 3, p 274.

Comment

Cardiac Masses

Thrombus is the most common cardiac or paracardiac mass. Among cardiac and paracardiac neoplasms, secondary tumors occur at 40 times the rate of primary neoplasms. Secondary tumors can involve the heart by direct extension (most commonly lymphoma or lymphadenopathy metastatic from lung or breast carcinoma) or by hematogenous spread (most commonly lung or breast carcinoma or melanoma). Primary benign tumors of the heart include myxoma, lipoma, and rhabdomyoma (associated with tuberous sclerosis). Primary malignant neoplasms include angiosarcoma and rhabdomyosarcoma.

Etiologies

Thrombi in the left ventricle are most commonly associated with an aneurysm. Coagulation disorders and flow abnormalities are less common causes of left ventricular thrombus.

Imaging Findings and Diagnostic Criteria

Echocardiography and CT can identify cardiac masses (Figs. A-C). MRI is the most accurate imaging examination for differentiation of tumor from thrombus. Neoplasms enhance homogeneously or heterogeneously after administration of gadolinium-chelate contrast agent, whereas bland thrombi typically do not enhance except in the periphery. On steady-state free precession (SSFP) MRI, a tumor usually shows intermediate signal intensity, and thrombus tends to demonstrate low signal intensity. However, myxomas can contain calcium and iron and can be dark on SSFP images.

Notes

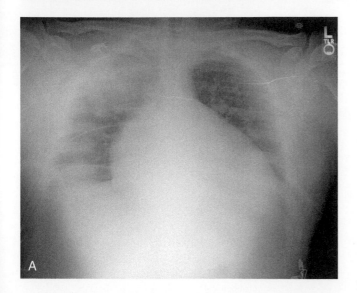

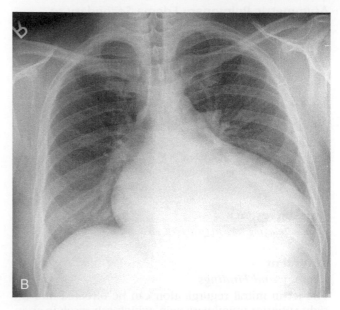

History: A patient presents with shortness of breath.

1. The radiograph in Fig. A was performed 1 month after the radiograph in Fig. B. What should be included in the differential diagnosis? (Choose all that apply.)
   A. Pneumonia
   B. Lung cancer
   C. Pulmonary edema
   D. Alveolar hemorrhage

2. What is the predominant distribution of the lung opacity?
   A. Right upper lobe
   B. Right lower lobe
   C. Left upper lobe
   D. Left lower lobe

3. If the patient had severe hemoptysis, what would be the most likely diagnosis?
   A. Pneumonia
   B. Lung cancer
   C. Pulmonary edema
   D. Alveolar hemorrhage

4. If the patient has mitral regurgitation, what is the most likely diagnosis?
   A. Pneumonia
   B. Lung cancer
   C. Pulmonary edema
   D. Alveolar hemorrhage

CASE 44

Asymmetric Pulmonary Edema Secondary to Mitral Regurgitation

1. A, C, and D

2. A

3. D

4. C

Reference

Walker CM, Reddy GP, Steiner RM: Radiology of the heart. In Rosendorff C, editor: *Essential Cardiology*, ed 3, Philadelphia, 2012, Saunders.

Cross-Reference

Cardiac Imaging: The REQUISITES, ed 3, p 23.

Comment

Etiology and Findings

The jet in mitral regurgitation can be directed into the right superior pulmonary vein, which can result in asymmetric right upper lobe pulmonary edema. Asymmetric right upper lobe pulmonary edema (Fig. A) is seen in 9% of adult patients and 22% of pediatric patients with severe mitral regurgitation. In adults, it is usually caused by a flail posterior valve leaflet secondary to myocardial infarction. A flail posterior leaflet causes the mitral regurgitant jet to be preferentially directed into the right superior pulmonary vein. This leads to focal increased hydrostatic pressure and pulmonary edema within the right upper lobe. In the setting of chest pain, acute mitral regurgitation must be considered and can be confirmed with echocardiography.

Differential Diagnosis

The differential diagnosis for right upper lobe opacity varies depending on the patient's clinical presentation. In a patient with fever and productive cough, the imaging findings are consistent with pneumonia. In a patient with hemoptysis, pulmonary hemorrhage is the most likely diagnosis. In a patient with severe chest pain and acute myocardial infarction, severe mitral regurgitation secondary to a flail posterior valve leaflet should be considered. If the abnormality has persisted over months, adenocarcinoma or organizing pneumonia must be excluded.

Notes

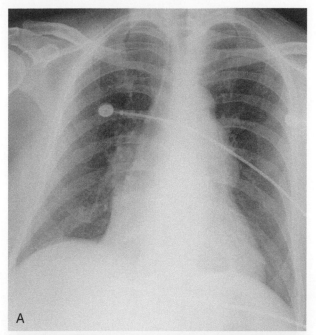

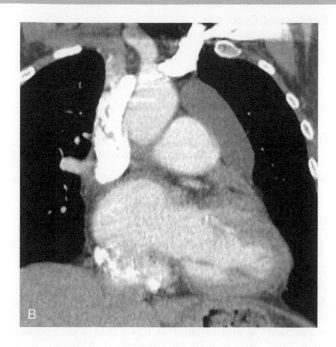

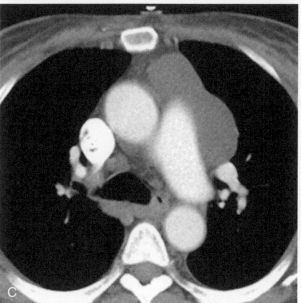

History: A patient presents with fever.

1. What should be included in the differential diagnosis based on the radiograph? (Choose all that apply.)
   A. Lymphoma
   B. Pericardial cyst
   C. Mitral stenosis
   D. Pulmonary stenosis

2. If the mass has a density of 8 HU, what is the most likely diagnosis?
   A. Thymoma
   B. Pericardial cyst
   C. Thymic cyst
   D. Lymphoma

3. What is the most common location of a pericardial cyst?
   A. Right cardiophrenic sulcus
   B. Left cardiophrenic sulcus
   C. Superior pericardial recess
   D. Subcarinal

4. Which of the following is least specific for a pericardial cyst?
   A. Hounsfield number of 10 on a non–contrast-enhanced CT image
   B. Hounsfield number of 30 on both a non–contrast-enhanced CT image and a contrast-enhanced CT image
   C. Low signal intensity on T1-weighted MRI
   D. High signal intensity on T2-weighted MRI

Pericardial Cyst

1. A, B, and D

2. B

3. A

4. C

References

Kim JS, Kim HH, Yoon Y: Imaging of pericardial diseases, *Clin Radiol* 62(7):626-631, 2007.

Wang ZJ, Reddy GP, Gotway MB, et al: CT and MR imaging of pericardial disease, *Radiographics* 23(Spec No):S167-S180, 2003.

Cross-Reference

Cardiac Imaging: The REQUISITES, ed 3, pp 78-79.

Comment

Etiology and Pathology

A pericardial cyst is a benign developmental lesion that is formed when a portion of the embryonic pericardium is pinched off and isolated. It has a thin wall, contains clear fluid, and is well circumscribed. The two most common locations are the right and left cardiophrenic angles. When a pericardial cyst is located in another area of the mediastinum, it can be difficult to differentiate from a bronchogenic, esophageal duplication, neuroenteric, or thymic cyst.

Imaging Features and Diagnosis

Radiographs typically show a nonspecific mediastinal contour abnormality (Fig. A). On CT and MRI, pericardial cysts are round or ovoid and are contiguous with the normal pericardium (Fig. B). CT shows a well-circumscribed mass (Fig. C). The density may be in the range of simple fluid, in which case the diagnosis is straightforward. If the density is higher, non–contrast-enhanced and contrast-enhanced CT can be performed to assess for enhancement. Pericardial cysts do not enhance, in contrast to neoplasms. Alternatively, MRI can be performed. On MRI, these lesions typically exhibit signal characteristics consistent with simple cysts found elsewhere in the body.

Notes

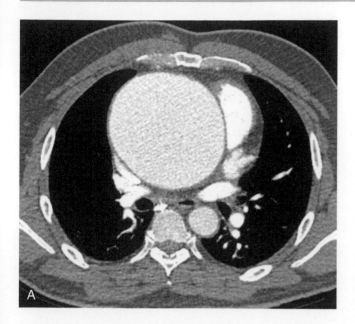

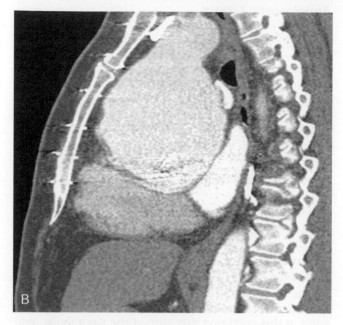

History: The patient is tall and thin.

1. What are some etiologies for this appearance?
   (Choose all that apply.)
   A. Marfan syndrome
   B. Atherosclerosis
   C. Syphilis
   D. Ehlers-Danlos syndrome

2. What is the most likely diagnosis?
   A. Marfan syndrome
   B. Atherosclerosis
   C. Syphilis
   D. Ehlers-Danlos syndrome

3. Which is the pathology of the aortic wall?
   A. Ruptured vasa vasorum
   B. Cystic medial necrosis
   C. Arteritis
   D. Atherosclerosis

4. What can be done to reduce the artifact resulting in
   the undulation of the anterior aortic wall seen in
   Fig. B?
   A. Dilution of contrast agent
   B. Dual energy
   C. Electrocardiogram gating
   D. Subtraction of calcium

Annuloaortic Ectasia

1. A and D

2. A

3. B

4. C

Reference

Reddy GP, Gunn M, Mitsumori LM, et al: Multislice CT and MRI of the thoracic aorta. In Webb WR, Higgins CB, editors: *Thoracic Imaging: Pulmonary and Cardiovascular Radiology*, ed 2, Philadelphia, 2010, Lippincott Williams & Wilkins.

Cross-Reference

Cardiac Imaging: The REQUISITES, ed 3, pp 388-389.

Comment

Pathology and Etiology

Enlargement of the aortic root and ascending aorta is characteristic of annuloaortic ectasia. The dilation of the aorta in this condition may stop at the sinotubular junction or extend to involve the entire ascending aorta, which is sometimes called the "tulip bulb" configuration. Annuloaortic ectasia results from cystic medial necrosis, which can be idiopathic or can be associated with Marfan syndrome or Ehlers-Danlos syndrome. Progression of annuloaortic ectasia in Marfan syndrome is generally more rapid than the idiopathic variant.

Complications

Complications of annuloaortic ectasia include aortic dissection, aortic rupture, and aortic regurgitation. Although 5.5 to 6 cm is the usual threshold of aortic diameter that necessitates surgery, operative repair may be indicated in annuloaortic ectasia when the aorta reaches a diameter of 5 cm or enlarges rapidly owing to the high risk of rupture.

Imaging

MRI and CT (Figs. A and B) are the most appropriate techniques for imaging of annuloaortic ectasia. MRI has the advantages of no ionizing radiation and the capability to provide quantitative assessment of aortic regurgitation.

Differential Diagnosis

Atherosclerosis is the leading cause of thoracic aortic aneurysms. Most atherosclerotic aneurysms occur in the descending thoracic aorta and commonly coexist with abdominal aortic aneurysms. Syphilis may cause ascending aortic aneurysms, but in contrast to annuloaortic ectasia, there is generally asymmetric involvement or no involvement of the sinuses of Valsalva and aortic root. Noninfectious arteritides (e.g., Takayasu arteritis, rheumatoid arthritis, giant cell arteritis) may cause thoracic aortic aneurysms. There is often circumferential aortic wall thickening with enhancement.

Notes

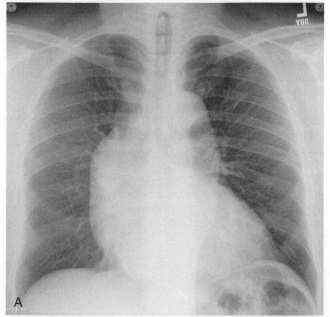

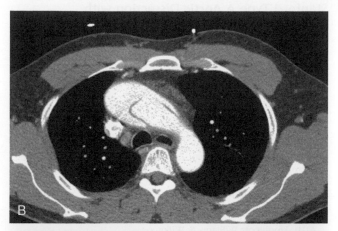

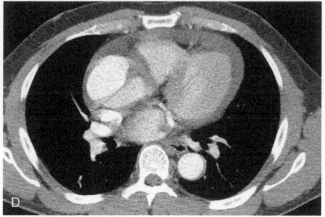

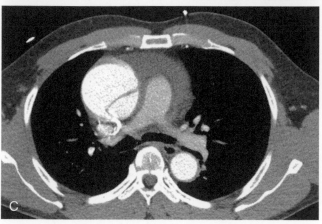

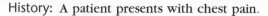

History: A patient presents with chest pain.

1. What are the causes of acute aortic syndrome?
   (Choose all that apply.)
   A. Penetrating ulcer
   B. Aneurysm
   C. Intramural hematoma
   D. Dissection

2. What is the most likely diagnosis?
   A. Intramural hematoma
   B. Penetrating aortic ulcer
   C. Aneurysm
   D. Dissection

3. What complication does this patient have?
   A. Coronary artery dissection
   B. Carotid artery dissection
   C. Acute aortic insufficiency
   D. Pericardial hemorrhage

4. What is the most appropriate management of this
   patient?
   A. No treatment
   B. Antihypertensive medication
   C. Close observation
   D. Surgery

Stanford Type A Aortic Dissection with Pericardial Hemorrhage

1. A, C, and D

2. D

3. D

4. D

References

Chin AS, Fleischmann D: State-of-the-art computed tomography angiography of acute aortic syndrome, *Semin Ultrasound CT MR* 33(3):222-234, 2012.

Reddy GP, Gunn M, Mitsumori LM, et al: Multislice CT and MRI of the thoracic aorta. In Webb WR, Higgins CB, editors: *Thoracic Imaging: Pulmonary and Cardiovascular Radiology*, ed 2, Philadelphia, 2010, Lippincott Williams & Wilkins.

Cross-Reference

Cardiac Imaging: The REQUISITES, ed 3, pp 378-387.

Comment

Acute Aortic Syndrome

Acute aortic syndrome is suspected in the setting of hypertension and chest pain radiating to the back. Acute aortic syndrome can be caused by aortic dissection, intramural hematoma, and penetrating aortic ulcer.

Etiology and Development

Aortic dissection is a separation of the aortic wall that results from intimal disruption. Blood can enter the aortic wall through a tear in the intima, extending proximally and distally in the media, displacing the intima inward. Typically, blood flows in both the true and the false lumina, although the false channel is sometimes thrombosed. The most common predisposing factor for aortic dissection is hypertension. Other etiologies include annuloaortic ectasia (which is associated with connective tissue disorders such as Marfan syndrome or Ehlers-Danlos syndrome), bicuspid aortic valve, aortic aneurysm, and arteritis.

Classification, Complications, and Management

Aortic dissection can be classified as Stanford type A (involving the ascending aorta) or type B (not involving the ascending aorta). The DeBakey classification system identifies three types of dissection: type I involves the ascending aorta and extends into the descending aorta; type II involves the ascending aorta only; and type III involves the descending aorta only, beyond the origin of the left subclavian artery. There are four major life-threatening complications of type A dissection: dissection of the coronary arteries resulting in myocardial infarction, dissection of the carotid arteries resulting in stroke, pericardial hemorrhage causing tamponade, and aortic valve rupture resulting in acute aortic regurgitation. Because of these potential complications, patients with type A dissection are usually treated surgically, with an ascending aortic graft. If the aortic valve is abnormal, the valve is replaced. In contrast, type B dissection usually can be managed medically, including the use of antihypertensive medications.

Imaging

Radiography can demonstrate aortic enlargement (Fig. A) and displacement of calcification; it has relatively low sensitivity and specificity for aortic dissection. CT has high accuracy for the diagnosis of aortic dissection and its complications (Figs. B-D). MRI has similar accuracy and can serve as an alternative imaging modality, especially when CT is contraindicated or in the setting of a chronic dissection. Transesophageal echocardiography (TEE) can be useful but may have lower specificity than CT or MRI. Even when it is not used to establish the diagnosis, TEE is often performed preoperatively to assess the status of the aortic valve.

Notes

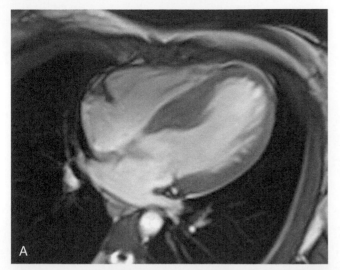

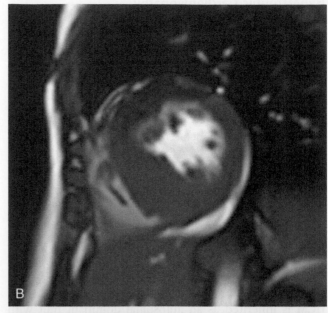

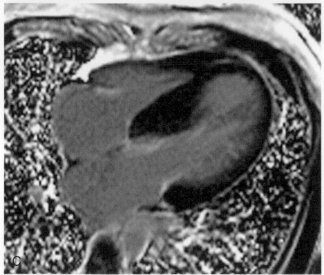

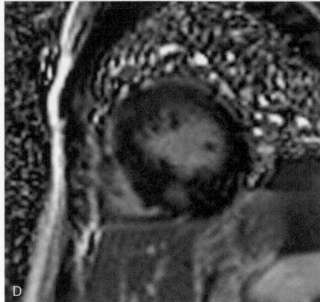

History: A 30-year-old woman presents with exercise-induced syncope.

1. What should be included in the differential diagnosis for this patient history? (Choose all that apply.)
   A. Arrhythmogenic right ventricular dysplasia
   B. Coronary artery anomaly
   C. Hypertrophic cardiomyopathy (HCM)
   D. Eisenmenger syndrome

2. Based on the images, what is the most likely diagnosis?
   A. Arrhythmogenic right ventricular dysplasia
   B. Coronary artery anomaly
   C. HCM
   D. Eisenmenger syndrome

3. What is the distribution of hypertrophy in this patient?
   A. Septal
   B. Concentric
   C. Midventricular
   D. Apical

4. Based on Fig. A, which of the following is in the differential diagnosis?
   A. Sarcoidosis
   B. Angiosarcoma
   C. Amyloidosis
   D. Hemochromatosis

CASE 48

Hypertrophic Cardiomyopathy

1. A, B, C, and D

2. C

3. A

4. B

References

Harris SR, Glockner J, Misselt AJ, et al: Cardiac MR imaging of nonisch-emic cardiomyopathies, *Magn Reson Imaging Clin N Am* 16(2):165-183, 2008.

Soler R, Rodriguez E, Remuinan C, et al: Magnetic resonance imaging of primary cardiomyopathies, *J Comput Assist Tomogr* 27(5):724-734, 2003.

Cross-Reference

Cardiac Imaging: The REQUISITES, ed 3, pp 53, 284–288.

Comment

Etiology and Clinical Features

HCM is inherited as an autosomal dominant trait with variable penetrance. Patients have a variable clinical presentation. They may be asymptomatic, or they may have atrial fibrillation, heart failure, syncope, or sudden cardiac death, which is the leading cause of mortality in these patients. Asymmetric hypertrophy of the ventricular septum accounts for 90% of cases of HCM. Other patterns exhibit right ventricular, left ventricular, septal, apical, midventricular, or concentric distribution. Patients with heart failure secondary to significant septal hypertrophy and left ventricular outflow obstruction can be treated with septal myectomy or percutaneous trans-luminal septal myocardial ablation with ethanol.

Imaging

MRI can provide anatomic and functional information in HCM and can be most useful when the diagnosis is in question, when invasive therapy is being considered, or when clinical concern requires more thorough assessment than that provided by echocardiography. MRI can be used to identify the distribution of thickened myocardium, to evaluate for systolic anterior motion of the mitral valve, and to calculate left ventricular mass (Figs. A-D). Late gadolinium enhancement MRI characteristically shows patchy midmyocardial enhancement. To differentiate HCM from a septal neoplasm, gadolinium-chelate contrast agent is administered intravenously. A neoplasm enhances markedly, whereas septal hypertrophic myocardium enhances only slightly. MRI also can be used for functional evaluation of left ventricular outflow tract obstruction and myocardial perfusion and viability.

Notes

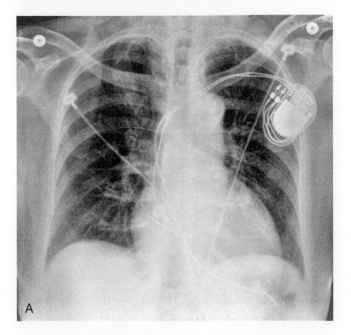

A

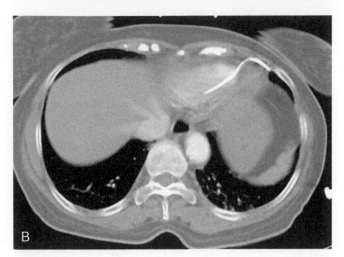

B

History: A 79-year-old woman presents with a malfunctioning pacemaker.

1. What are causes of pacemaker malfunction? (Choose all that apply.)
   A. Lead fracture
   B. Disconnection of lead from generator
   C. Lead dislodgment
   D. Lead perforation

2. What is the most likely diagnosis?
   A. Lead fracture
   B. Disconnection of lead from generator
   C. Lead dislodgment
   D. Lead perforation

3. Where is the lead that is to the left of midline?
   A. Right ventricle
   B. Coronary sinus
   C. Left ventricle
   D. Outside of the heart

4. Where is the lead that is to the right of midline?
   A. Right atrium
   B. Right ventricle
   C. Left atrium
   D. Superior vena cava

Perforation of Pacemaker Lead

1. A, B, C, and D

2. D

3. D

4. A

Reference

Aguilera AL, Volokhina YV, Fisher KL: Radiography of cardiac conduction devices: a comprehensive review, *Radiographics* 31(6):1669–1682, 2011.

Comment

Normal Appearance of Pacemakers

Cardiac pacemakers are used in patients with conduction disturbances. Types of pacemakers include single chamber (pacing the right ventricle or right atrium), dual chamber (pacing both the right atrium and right ventricle), and biventricular (pacing the right atrium, right ventricle, and left ventricle). Biventricular pacing is also called cardiac resynchronization therapy. Patients often have combined pacemaker and implantable cardioverter-defibrillators (ICDs). An ICD is used to defibrillate the heart during a potentially fatal arrhythmia and is distinguished from a pacemaker lead by its thick radiopaque shock coil.

Complications of Pacemakers

Acute complications of pacemaker placement include pneumothorax, hemothorax, arrhythmia secondary to inappropriate lead placement, and myocardial perforation. In the setting of long-term pacemaker placement, complications include lead disconnection from the generator, lead fracture, lead displacement, and perforation. Twiddler syndrome is a unique form of lead displacement caused by the conscious or subconscious rotating of the generator in the subcutaneous tissues by the patient. It may be recognized on radiography by noting lead displacement with leads curled around the generator.

Imaging Findings and Diagnostic Criteria

Chest radiography can be used to identify disruption of the lead, migration, and perforation (Fig. A). When additional information is needed, CT scan may be performed (Fig. B).

Notes

Fair Game

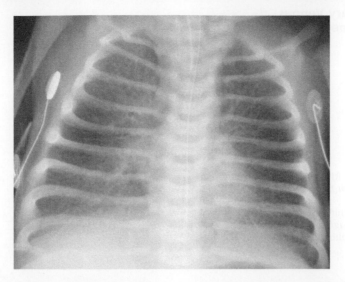

History: A 1-day-old neonate has shortness of breath.

1. What should be included in the differential
diagnosis for pulmonary edema in an infant?
(Choose all that apply.)
A. Tetralogy of Fallot
B. Coarctation of the aorta
C. Vein of Galen malformation
D. Total anomalous pulmonary venous connection

2. What is the finding seen on the chest radiograph?
A. Cardiomegaly
B. Pulmonary edema
C. Pleural effusions
D. Right aortic arch

3. What is the most likely diagnosis in this patient?
A. Tetralogy of Fallot
B. Coarctation of the aorta
C. Vein of Galen malformation
D. Total anomalous pulmonary venous connection

4. Which type of total anomalous pulmonary venous
connection is most likely to manifest with a
"snowman heart" configuration on chest
radiography?
A. Supracardiac
B. Cardiac
C. Infracardiac
D. Mixed

Total Anomalous Pulmonary Venous Connection Type III (Connection below Diaphragm)

1. B, C, and D

2. B

3. D

4. A

References

Dillman JR, Yarram SG, Hernandez RJ: Imaging of pulmonary venous developmental anomalies, *AJR Am J Roentgenol* 192(5):1272-1285, 2009.

Higgins CB: Radiography of congenital heart disease. In Webb WR, Higgins CB, editors: *Thoracic imaging: Pulmonary and cardiovascular radiology*, ed 2, Philadelphia, 2010, Lippincott Williams & Wilkins.

Cross-Reference

Cardiac Imaging: The REQUISITES, ed 3, pp 328-330.

Comment

Types of Total Anomalous Pulmonary Venous Connection

In this anomaly, all the pulmonary veins drain into the systemic veins or directly into the right atrium. In the supracardiac type (type I), the enlarged mediastinal veins cause the "snowman heart" appearance. In the cardiac type (type II), the pulmonary veins drain into the coronary sinus or right atrium. In the infracardiac type (type III), the veins connect to the portal vein, hepatic vein, or ductus venosus. Venous flow is obstructed by the passage of the pulmonary veins across the esophageal hiatus, leading to pulmonary congestion and edema without cardiac enlargement.

Radiography

The chest radiograph typically shows shunt vascularity. In total anomalous pulmonary venous connection type III (connection below the diaphragm), the radiograph shows pulmonary edema with a normal-sized heart (Figure).

Notes

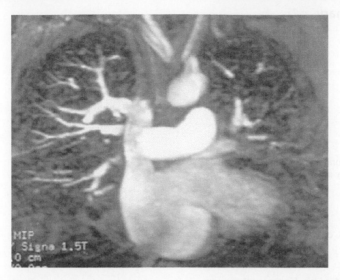

History: A patient presents with pulmonary hypertension.

1. What shunt lesions can cause pulmonary hypertension?
   A. Atrial septal defect (ASD)
   B. Ventricular septal defect (VSD)
   C. Patent ductus arteriosus (PDA)
   D. Partial anomalous pulmonary venous connection (PAPVC)

2. What is the most likely diagnosis?
   A. ASD
   B. VSD
   C. PDA
   D. PAPVC

3. Which lesion is commonly associated with this anomaly?
   A. VSD
   B. ASD
   C. PDA
   D. Truncus arteriosus

4. Which other lesion is most physiologically similar to PAPVC?
   A. VSD
   B. ASD
   C. PDA
   D. Aorticopulmonary window (septal defect)

CASE 51

Partial Anomalous Pulmonary Venous Connection

1. A, B, C, and D

2. D

3. B

4. B

Reference

Reddy GP, Higgins CB: Magnetic resonance imaging of congenital heart disease: evaluation of morphology and function, *Semin Roentgenol* 38(4):342-351, 2003.

Cross-Reference

Cardiac Imaging: The REQUISITES, ed 3, pp 330-335.

Comment

Physiology and Associated Anomalies

Depending on the severity of the shunt, patients with PAPVC may be asymptomatic; may have dyspnea, cardiac murmur, and decreased exercise tolerance; or may have pulmonary hypertension. Because it is an atrial-level shunt, PAPVC is physiologically similar to ASD. PAPVC is associated with other congenital abnormalities, most commonly a sinus venosus ASD, in which a connection exists between the left atrium and the superior vena cava as the cava enters the right atrium.

Imaging

Medical and surgical management depends on accurate evaluation of the number and site of anomalous pulmonary veins and the presence of an ASD or other congenital anomaly. Gadolinium-enhanced magnetic resonance angiography (MRA) can accurately depict the presence, location, and size of anomalous veins in patients with PAPVC (Figure). MRI has the advantage over CT and angiography of no ionizing radiation or iodinated contrast agent.

Notes

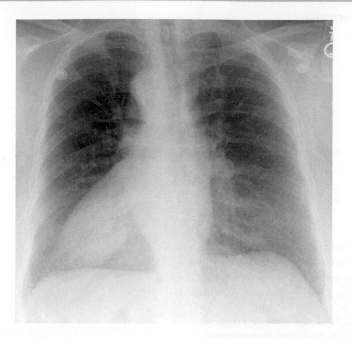

History: No patient history is available.

1. Which findings are present? (Choose all that apply.)
   A. Dextrocardia
   B. Right aortic arch
   C. Liver on right
   D. Stomach on left

2. What is the most likely diagnosis?
   A. Situs solitus with levocardia
   B. Situs solitus with dextrocardia
   C. Situs inversus with levocardia
   D. Situs inversus with dextrocardia

3. Which large airway disease is associated with this anomaly?
   A. Cystic fibrosis
   B. Tracheobronchomegaly
   C. Immotile cilia syndrome
   D. Allergic bronchopulmonary aspergillosis

4. What percentage of patients with situs inversus totalis have congenital heart disease?
   A. 1% to 2%
   B. 5% to 10%
   C. 40% to 50%
   D. 90% to 95%

CASE 52

Situs Inversus with Dextrocardia

1. A and B

2. D

3. C

4. B

Reference

Spoon JM: Situs inversus totalis, *Neonatal Netw* 20(1):59–63, 2001.

Cross-Reference

Cardiac Imaging: The REQUISITES, ed 3, p 302.

Comment

Clinical Information and Associated Anomalies

Most individuals who have situs inversus totalis can live into adulthood without intervention. There is an association with Kartagener (immotile cilia) syndrome, in which patients have bronchiectasis, sinusitis, and infertility. Only 5% to 10% of these individuals have a congenital cardiac lesion. Situs ambiguus (visceral heterotaxy) or situs solitus with dextrocardia is strongly associated with complex congenital heart disease. There are two major types of situs ambiguus or heterotaxia: bilateral right-sidedness (asplenia syndrome) and bilateral left-sidedness (polysplenia syndrome). Patients with asplenia syndrome generally present early in life with cyanosis and complex congenital heart disease (e.g., transposition of the great arteries, double outlet right ventricle, common atrioventricular valve). Patients with polysplenia syndrome present later in life with less severe congenital heart defects (e.g., atrial septal defect, partial anomalous pulmonary venous connection).

Imaging

Imaging is usually straightforward; chest radiographs show that the cardiac apex is on the right and the abdominal viscera are inverted (Figure). For a complete diagnosis, CT, MRI, or cineangiography can be used to identify the left-sided inferior vena cava entering the anatomic right atrium and the left-sided liver. Dextrocardia should be differentiated from dextroversion. In dextroversion, the heart is simply shifted to the right but the cardiac apex and stomach bubble remain directed towards the left. Causes of dextroversion include the Scimitar syndrome or left-sided masses such as congenital diaphragmatic hernia.

Notes

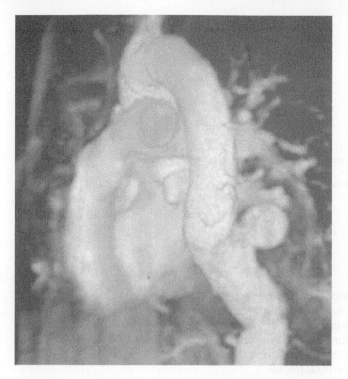

History: A patient presents with chest pain.

1. What are potential etiologies of this abnormality? (Choose all that apply.)
   A. Marfan syndrome
   B. Atherosclerosis
   C. Infection
   D. Trauma

2. Which portion of the aorta is most abnormal?
   A. Ascending
   B. Arch
   C. Descending
   D. Abdominal

3. What is the most likely diagnosis?
   A. True aneurysm
   B. Pseudoaneurysm
   C. Aortic diverticulum
   D. Intramural hematoma

4. What type of image is shown?
   A. Volume rendering
   B. Curved multiplanar reformation
   C. Maximum intensity projection
   D. Minimum intensity projection

Mycotic Pseudoaneurysm

1. B, C, and D

2. C

3. B

4. A

Reference

Reddy GP, Gunn M, Mitsumori LM, et al: Multislice CT and MRI of the thoracic aorta. In Webb WR, Higgins CB, editors: *Thoracic imaging: pulmonary and cardiovascular radiology*, ed 2, Philadelphia, 2010, Lippincott Williams & Wilkins.

Cross-Reference

Cardiac Imaging: The REQUISITES, ed 3, pp 377-379.

Comment

Etiology and Pathology

Etiologies of aortic pseudoaneurysm include atherosclerosis (penetrating aortic ulcer), infection, trauma (deceleration injury—although this is an unusual location), and iatrogenic cause. Pseudoaneurysms are characterized by disruption of one or more layers of the vessel wall, whereas true aneurysms have intact walls.

True and False Aneurysm

In a true aneurysm of the aorta, all three layers of the aortic wall are intact. In contrast, a false aneurysm results from a focal disruption of one or more layers of the aortic wall and may be contained by the adventitia and surrounding fibrous tissue.

Imaging

CT and MRI are the best imaging methods for evaluation of a thoracic aortic aneurysm. Disruption of the wall is difficult to identify on imaging. However, many observers use the following rule of thumb: a relatively narrow ostium (<50% of the aneurysm diameter) suggests that the outpouching is a pseudoaneurysm (Figure), and a wide ostium suggests a true aneurysm.

Notes

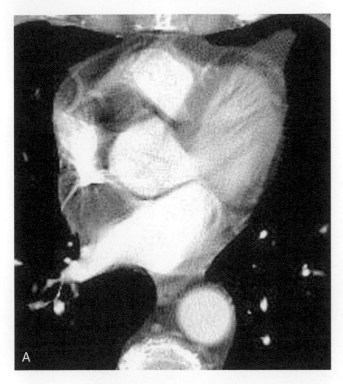

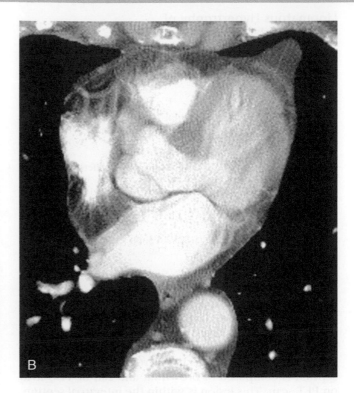

History: A patient with lung cancer has a fluorode-oxyglucose (FDG)-avid mass seen on PET/CT scan.

1. Which chambers are most closely associated with the mass? (Choose all that apply.)
   A. Left atrium
   B. Left ventricle
   C. Right atrium
   D. Right ventricle

2. Where is the mass located?
   A. Left atrium
   B. Right atrium
   C. Interatrial septum
   D. Aortic root

3. What is the most likely diagnosis?
   A. Lipoma
   B. Lipomatous hypertrophy
   C. Pericardial cyst
   D. Metastasis

4. Why is the mass FDG avid?
   A. It represents a metastasis.
   B. It represents an angiosarcoma.
   C. It is composed of brown fat.
   D. The PET and CT images were not correctly aligned.

Lipomatous Hypertrophy of the Interatrial Septum

1. A and C

2. C

3. B

4. C

Reference

Maurer AH, Burshteyn M, Adler LP, et al: How to differentiate benign versus malignant cardiac and paracardiac 18F FDG uptake at oncologic PET/CT, *Radiographics* 31(5):1287–1305, 2011.

Cross-Reference

Cardiac Imaging: The REQUISITES, ed 3, pp 149, 282.

Comment

Clinical Features

Lipomatous hypertrophy of the interatrial septum is benign and is characterized by fat in the interatrial septum. It occurs more frequently in elderly, obese patients and is associated with an increased amount of epicardial fat. Lipomatous hypertrophy of the interatrial septum is composed of brown fat and can be FDG avid on PET scan. This lesion is within the interatrial septum, not in the atrium, and it does not normally need to be resected.

Imaging

The lesion is sometimes seen on echocardiography or PET scan, and patients are referred to CT or MRI to differentiate intraatrial lipoma or thrombus from lipomatous hypertrophy (Figs. A and B). In other instances, the mass is discovered incidentally on CT or MRI. When MRI is performed, fat saturation images can confirm the composition of the mass. The mass can have a narrow waist in the region of the fossa ovalis.

Notes

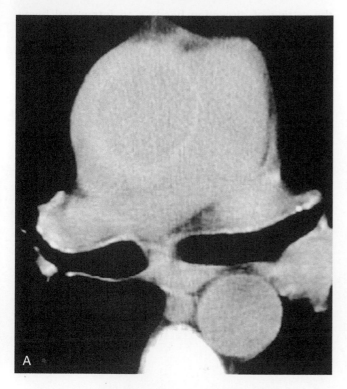

A

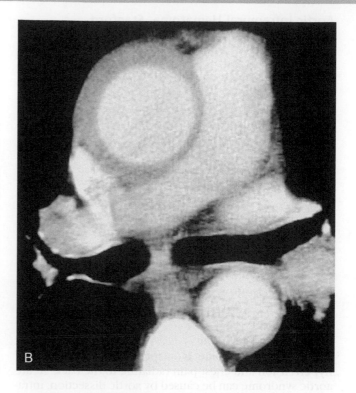

B

History: A patient presents with chest pain.

1. What are the causes of acute aortic syndrome?
   (Choose all that apply.)
   A. Aneurysm
   B. Dissection
   C. Intramural hematoma
   D. Penetrating ulcer

2. What is the most likely diagnosis?
   A. Aneurysm
   B. Dissection
   C. Intramural hematoma
   D. Penetrating ulcer

3. What is the most likely cause of this finding?
   A. Rupture of the vasa vasorum
   B. Communication with the aortic lumen
   C. Trauma
   D. Venous bleeding

4. Which of the following is *not* an appropriate
   management of this patient?
   A. No treatment
   B. Antihypertensive medication
   C. Close observation
   D. Surgery

Aortic Intramural Hematoma, Stanford Type A

1. B, C, and D

2. C

3. A

4. A

References

Chin AS, Fleischmann D: State-of-the-art computed tomography angiography of acute aortic syndrome, *Semin Ultrasound CT MR* 33(3):222-234, 2012.

Reddy GP, Gunn M, Mitsumori LM, et al: Multislice CT and MRI of the thoracic aorta. In Webb WR, Higgins CB, editors: *Thoracic imaging: pulmonary and cardiovascular radiology*, ed 2, Philadelphia, 2010, Lippincott Williams & Wilkins.

Cross-Reference

Cardiac Imaging: The REQUISITES, ed 3, p 411.

Comment

Acute Aortic Syndrome

Acute aortic syndrome is suspected in the setting of hypertension and chest pain radiating to the back. Acute aortic syndrome can be caused by aortic dissection, intramural hematoma, and penetrating aortic ulcer.

Etiology and Management

An intramural hematoma is most commonly caused by rupture of the vasa vasorum, the arteries that supply the aortic wall. The ruptured vessels bleed into the aortic wall, which can result in an intimal tear and separation of the wall—a classic dissection. If the intima does not separate, an intramural hematoma remains. The intramural hematoma may remain localized, or it can extend along the wall in an antegrade or a retrograde direction or rarely rupture through the adventitia. Intramural hematoma can be considered to be a type of dissection, and treatment is similar to treatment of a frank dissection. Stanford type B intramural hematoma (not involving the ascending aorta) is usually managed medically. Traditionally, type A intramural hematoma (not involving the ascending aorta) is treated with surgery. In recent years, some surgeons have begun to manage type A hematoma conservatively with antihypertensive medication and close observation. Patients who develop pericardial hemorrhage, aortic valve regurgitation, or extension of hematoma into the coronary or arch vessels need surgery.

Imaging

Non–contrast-enhanced CT scan shows characteristic high-density thickening of the aortic wall, indicating intramural hematoma (Fig. A). Contrast-enhanced CT scan shows the thickening of the wall, but the high density may be difficult to appreciate (Fig. B). On MRI, the signal intensity is intermediate to high on black blood sequences. Relying solely on gadolinium-enhanced magnetic resonance angiography (MRA) can be risky in the setting of dissection because an intramural hematoma can be overlooked on this sequence.

Notes

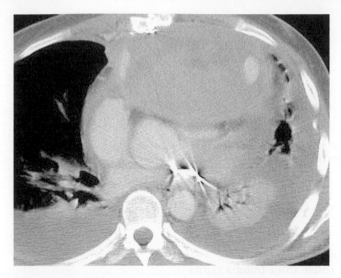

History: A patient presents with chest pain.

1. What should be included in the differential diagnosis? (Choose all that apply.)
   A. Cyst
   B. Lipoma
   C. Metastasis
   D. Hematoma

2. What is the most likely location of the mass?
   A. Pericardium
   B. Myocardium
   C. Right ventricle
   D. Left ventricle

3. What is the most likely diagnosis?
   A. Cyst
   B. Lipoma
   C. Metastasis
   D. Hematoma

4. Which chamber is most severely compressed?
   A. Left atrium
   B. Left ventricle
   C. Right atrium
   D. Right ventricle

Pericardial Hematoma

1. C and D

2. A

3. D

4. D

Reference

Wang ZJ, Reddy GP, Gotway MB, et al: CT and MR imaging of pericardial disease, *Radiographics* 23(Spec No):S167–S180, 2003.

Cross-Reference

Cardiac Imaging: The REQUISITES, ed 3, pp 265, 270.

Comment

Etiology and Physiology

A pericardial hematoma can result from trauma (iatrogenic or otherwise), myocardial infarction, aortic dissection, tumor, or pericarditis. When a hematoma is large enough to compress a cardiac chamber and cause hemodynamic compromise, it may have to be evacuated to relieve the compression.

Differential Diagnosis

The differential diagnosis for a pericardial mass includes a pericardial cyst, tumor (metastatic or primary), and hematoma.

1. Pericardial cysts are of water attenuation on CT and are hyperintense on T2-weighted MRI. They do not enhance following contrast administration. Occasionally pericardial cysts are hyperdense on CT or have high intrinsic T1 signal when they contain proteinaceous fluid.

2. Primary and metastatic tumors cause hemopericardium and pericardial nodules or masses. Unlike pericardial cyst and hematoma, tumor enhances following contrast administration. Most pericardial tumors are secondary to direct extension or hematogenous spread from lung or breast carcinoma, lymphoma, and melanoma. Primary pericardial tumors are rare; mesothelioma is the most common. Other primary pericardial tumors include lymphoma and teratoma.

3. Pericardial hematoma is characterized by high or heterogeneous density on CT (Figure). A chronic hematoma can be calcified. MRI is useful as it may show characteristic high T1 and T2 signal from associated blood product degradation. Hematomas do not enhance following contrast administration.

Notes

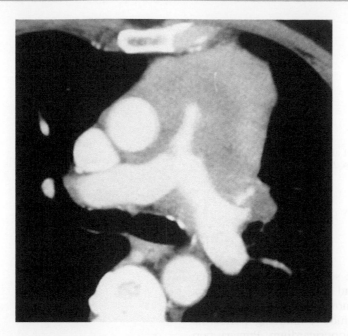

History: A patient presents with shortness of breath.

1. What should be included in the differential diagnosis? (Choose all that apply.)
   A. Breast cancer metastasis
   B. Lung cancer metastasis
   C. Melanoma metastasis
   D. Lymphoma

2. Which structure is most severely compressed?
   A. Pulmonary artery
   B. Aorta
   C. Bronchus
   D. Superior vena cava

3. What is the most likely diagnosis?
   A. Secondary tumor
   B. Primary benign tumor
   C. Primary malignant tumor
   D. Hematoma

4. What is the most likely location of the mass?
   A. Pulmonary artery
   B. Anterior mediastinum
   C. Myocardium
   D. Pericardium

Pericardial Lymphoma

1. A, B, C, and D

2. A

3. A

4. D

Reference

Yared K, Baggish AL, Picard MH, et al: Multimodality imaging of pericardial diseases, *JACC Cardiovasc Imaging* 3(6):650–660, 2010.

Cross-Reference

Cardiac Imaging: The REQUISITES, ed 3, pp 102–104.

Comment

Radiographic Features

Most pericardial tumors are secondary to direct extension or hematogenous spread from lung or breast carcinoma, lymphoma, and melanoma. Findings suggestive of pericardial malignancy include enhancing pericardial nodules or masses and hemopericardium. Primary pericardial tumors are rare; mesothelioma is the most common. Other primary pericardial tumors include lymphoma and teratoma.

Primary Cardiac Lymphoma

Primary pericardial lymphoma is associated with acquired immunodeficiency syndrome (AIDS) and is generally a non-Hodgkin lymphoma. By definition, the lymphoma is localized to the heart or pericardium at diagnosis without evidence of systemic disease. Presenting symptoms include rapidly progressive heart failure, arrhythmia, cardiac tamponade, superior vena cava syndrome, and chest pain. Pleural effusion, including hemorrhagic effusion, occurs frequently. The prognosis of primary cardiac lymphoma is poor with many patients being diagnosed at autopsy. Treatment includes chemotherapy and tumor debulking for palliative control of symptoms.

Imaging

CT is frequently performed for diagnosis, but MRI is especially useful to define the extent of involvement. Lymphoma is typically infiltrative and follows the pericardial contour (Figure). Both CT and MRI show heterogeneous enhancement following the administration of intravenous contrast. Cross-sectional imaging plays an important role in assessing disease response to therapy.

Notes

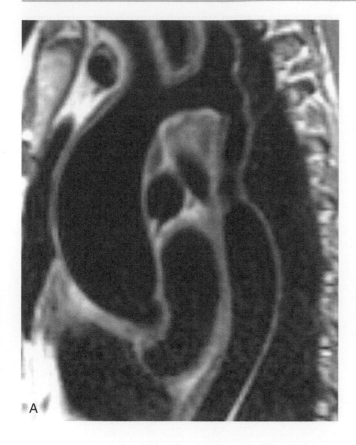

A

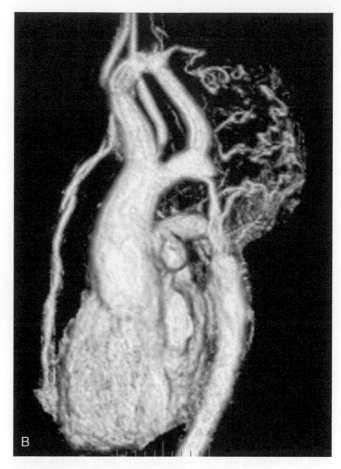

B

History: A patient presents with hypertension.

1. What should be included in the differential diagnosis? (Choose all that apply.)
   A. Coarctation of the aorta
   B. Kawasaki disease
   C. Giant cell arteritis
   D. Takayasu arteritis

2. Which portion of the aorta is narrowed?
   A. Ascending
   B. Arch
   C. Descending
   D. Abdominal

3. What is the most likely diagnosis?
   A. Coarctation of the aorta
   B. Kawasaki disease
   C. Giant cell arteritis
   D. Takayasu arteritis

4. Which MRI sequence can be used to quantify collateral circulation?
   A. Contrast-enhanced magnetic resonance angiography (MRA)
   B. Steady-state free precession (SSFP)
   C. Velocity-encoded cine phase contrast
   D. Late gadolinium enhancement inversion recovery

Takayasu Arteritis—Long-Segment Coarctation

1. A, C, and D

2. C

3. D

4. C

References

Gotway MB, Araoz PA, Macedo TA, et al: Imaging findings in Takayasu's arteritis, *AJR Am J Roentgenol* 184(6):1945-1950, 2005.

Hom JJ, Ordovas K, Reddy GP: Velocity-encoded cine MR imaging in aortic coarctation: functional assessment of hemodynamic events, *Radiographics* 28(2):407-416, 2008.

Reddy GP, Gunn M, Mitsumori LM, et al: Multislice CT and MRI of the thoracic aorta. In Webb WR, Higgins CB, editors: *Thoracic imaging: pulmonary and cardiovascular radiology*, ed 2, Philadelphia, 2010, Lippincott Williams & Wilkins.

Cross-Reference

Cardiac Imaging: The REQUISITES, ed 3, pp 393-394.

Comment

Clinical Features

Congenital coarctation is most commonly discrete and juxtaductal in location. Long-segment coarctations may be acquired; Takayasu arteritis is an important cause. Takayasu arteritis (pulseless disease or Martorell syndrome) is an idiopathic disease that is characterized by wall thickening of the aorta and/or arch vessels along with stenosis of the aorta and its branches. Other arteries, such as the pulmonary arteries, can be involved. Patients typically have nonspecific systemic symptoms during the active phase of the disease. In the sclerotic phase, symptoms of vascular insufficiency develop, including abdominal angina and claudication. Hypertension is frequent. The two main large vessel arteritidies include Takayasu and giant cell arteritis which are differentiated by clinical features. Takayasu arteritis most commonly affects women between 10 and 40 years of age, whereas giant cell arteritis occurs in patients older than 50. High-dose corticosteroids are generally the treatment of choice.

Imaging

In Takayasu arteritis, MRI and CT can show stenosis, occlusion, or dilation of the aorta and its branches or a combination of all three. On MRI, the active phase of the disease manifests as wall thickening and enhancement. An aortic wall thickness of greater than 3 mm has been proposed as a marker for early Takayasu arteritis. In the sclerotic phase, MRI can demonstrate areas of stenosis (Figs. A and B) and CT can show concentric aortic wall calcification. Velocity-encoded cine phase contrast imaging can be used to measure collateral circulation. PET is useful for monitoring disease response in patients with large vessel vasculitides. Decreasing FDG activity is considered a favorable response to therapy and may be seen prior to anatomic imaging showing decreased aortic wall thickening.

Notes

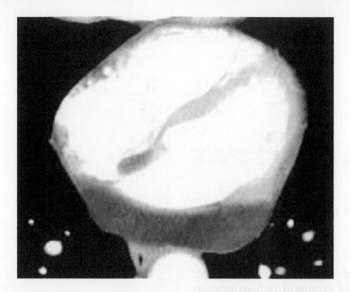

History: A patient presents with retroperitoneal liposarcoma.

1. What should be included in the differential diagnosis? (Choose all that apply.)
   A. Cyst
   B. Lipoma
   C. Metastasis
   D. Hematoma

2. What is the most likely location of the mass?
   A. Pericardium
   B. Myocardium
   C. Left atrium
   D. Right atrium

3. What is the most likely diagnosis?
   A. Cyst
   B. Lipoma
   C. Metastasis
   D. Hematoma

4. What is the most appropriate management?
   A. No treatment
   B. Chemotherapy
   C. Radiation therapy
   D. Surgery

CASE 59

Pericardial Lipoma

1. B and C

2. A

3. B

4. A

Reference

Yared K, Baggish AL, Picard MH, et al: Multimodality imaging of peri-cardial diseases, *JACC Cardiovasc Imaging* 3(6):650–660, 2010.

Cross-Reference

Cardiac Imaging: The REQUISITES, ed 3, p 273.

Comment

Clinical Features

Cardiac lipoma most commonly occurs in the right atrium. It is the second most common benign primary cardiac neoplasm following myxoma. Other locations include the epicardium, endocardium, interatrial septum, and left ventricle. Pericardial lipomas are less common, but they are among the more common masses of the pericardium. Lipomas tend to be soft and flexible, and even large tumors may not compress the heart. They are usually asymptomatic. If there are symptoms of compression, such as pain or shortness of breath, then surgical resection is usually performed.

CT and MRI Features

On CT scan, a pericardial lipoma manifests as a homogeneous, low-density mass (negative Hounsfield units) in the pericardium that is relatively pliable without much mass effect (Figure). There is generally no enhancement and no signs of invasion. Fat saturation MRI sequences are ideal for demonstrating that the mass is composed of fat.

Associations

Multiple fat-containing masses within the myocardium have been described in patients with tuberous sclerosis. Current pathologic literature suggests these fatty lesions may simply represent unencapsulated fat cells rather than true encapsulated cardiac lipomas.

Notes

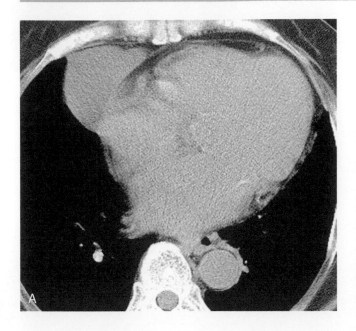

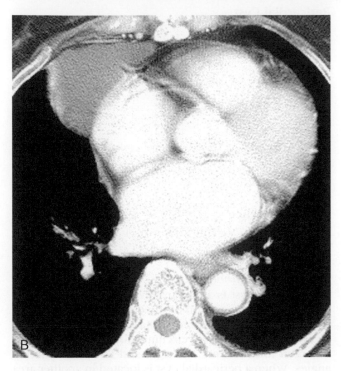

History: A patient has a cardiophrenic angle mass on chest radiography.

1. What should be included in the differential diagnosis based on Fig. A, in which the mass measures 35 HU? (Choose all that apply.)
   A. Fat pad
   B. Pericardial cyst
   C. Metastasis
   D. Lymphoma

2. What is the most likely diagnosis based on Figs. A and B? The mass measures 35 HU in Fig. A and 36 HU in Fig. B.
   A. Fat pad
   B. Pericardial cyst
   C. Metastasis
   D. Lymphoma

3. What is the most common presentation of a pericardial cyst?
   A. Asymptomatic
   B. Pain
   C. Shortness of breath
   D. Fever

4. What is the most appropriate management of this mass?
   A. No treatment
   B. Chemotherapy
   C. Radiation therapy
   D. Surgery

Pericardial Cyst

1. B, C, and D

2. B

3. A

4. A

References

Kim JS, Kim HH, Yoon Y: Imaging of pericardial diseases, *Clin Radiol* 62(7):626-631, 2007.

Wang ZJ, Reddy GP, Gotway MB, et al: CT and MR imaging of pericardial disease, *Radiographics* 23(Spec No):S167-S180, 2003.

Cross-Reference

Cardiac Imaging: The REQUISITES, ed 3, pp 78-79

Comment

Etiology and Pathology

A pericardial cyst is a benign developmental lesion that is formed when a portion of the embryonic pericardium is pinched off and isolated. It has a thin wall, contains clear fluid, and is well circumscribed. The two most common locations are the right and left cardiophrenic angles. When a pericardial cyst is located in another area of the mediastinum, it can be difficult to differentiate from a bronchogenic, esophageal duplication, neuroenteric, or thymic cyst. Pericardial cysts are usually homogeneous and well circumscribed. Often they contain simple fluid, but they can contain complex hemorrhagic or proteinaceous fluid.

Imaging Features and Diagnosis

On CT and MRI, pericardial cysts are round or ovoid and are contiguous with the normal pericardium. CT shows a well-circumscribed mass (Figs. A and B). The density may be in the range of simple fluid, in which case the diagnosis is straightforward. If the density is higher, noncontrast and contrast-enhanced CT scans can be performed to assess for enhancement (Figs. A and B). Pericardial cysts do not enhance, in contrast to neoplasms. Alternatively, MRI can be performed. On MRI, these lesions typically exhibit signal characteristics consistent with simple cysts found elsewhere in the body. They appear as low to intermediate signal masses on T1-weighted images (Fig. B) and high signal intensity lesions on T2-weighted images.

Notes

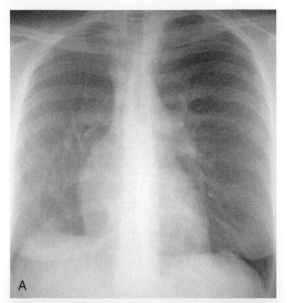

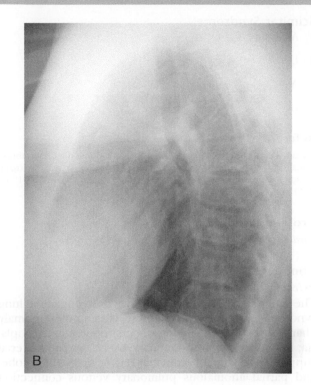

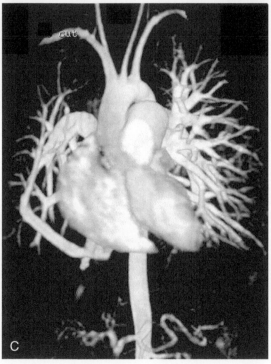

History: A patient presents with easy fatigability.

1. What lesions are likely present in this patient?
   (Choose all that apply.)
   A. Hypoplastic right lung
   B. Hypoplastic right pulmonary artery
   C. Hypoplastic right main bronchus
   D. Hypoplastic right atrium

2. What is the most common shunt lesion in this anomaly?
   A. Atrial septal defect
   B. Ventricular septal defect
   C. Patent ductus arteriosus
   D. Partial anomalous pulmonary venous connection

3. Where do the anomalous pulmonary veins drain?
   A. Inferior vena cava
   B. Superior vena cava
   C. Coronary sinus
   D. Portal vein

4. What is the most likely diagnosis?
   A. Agenesis of the right lung
   B. Scimitar syndrome
   C. Total anomalous pulmonary venous connection
   D. Proximal interruption of the right pulmonary artery

CASE 61

Scimitar Syndrome

1. A, B, and C

2. D

3. A

4. B

Reference

Biyyam DR, Chapman T, Ferguson MR, et al: Congenital lung abnormalities: embryologic features, prenatal diagnosis, and postnatal radiologic-pathologic correlation, *Radiographics* 30(6):1721–1738, 2010.

Cross-Reference

Cardiac Imaging: The REQUISITES, ed 3, pp 334–336.

Comment

Primary Anomalies

The scimitar syndrome, also known as hypogenetic lung syndrome or venolobar syndrome, is a complex anomaly characterized by four components: right lung hypoplasia; hypoplastic right pulmonary artery; systemic arterial supply (from the abdominal aorta) of right lower lobe; and partial anomalous pulmonary venous connection from the right lung, most commonly into the inferior vena cava or occasionally into the right atrium, portal vein, azygos vein, or a hepatic vein. All four components need not be present to make the diagnosis. The name scimitar syndrome arises from the anomalous pulmonary vein, which can have the appearance of a scimitar, a curved Turkish sword.

Associated Anomalies

Associated findings include hypoplastic right bronchus or other abnormalities of the tracheobronchial tree and cardiac anomalies such as atrial septal defect. The partial anomalous pulmonary venous connection in scimitar syndrome is a left-to-right shunt at the atrial level, with physiology similar to an atrial septal defect. The severity of the shunt has a substantial effect on the clinical course.

Imaging

Chest radiography (Figs. A and B), echocardiography, and cineangiography have been used to establish the diagnosis. In recent years, MRI has been used as a non-invasive means of diagnosis. Gadolinium-enhanced MRA can be used to demonstrate the anomalous venous drainage, the hypoplastic ipsilateral pulmonary artery, and the systemic arterial supply to the right lung base (Fig. C). Velocity-encoded phase contrast cine MRI can be used to assess cardiac function in scimitar syndrome by quantifying the degree of left-to-right shunting and by differentiating left and right pulmonary arterial blood flow.

Notes

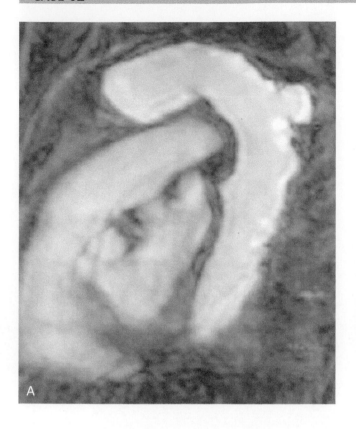

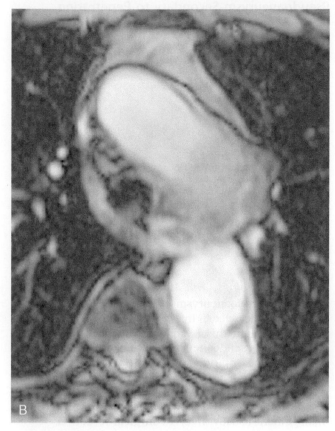

History: A patient presents with chest pain.

1. What are the causes of acute aortic syndrome?
   (Choose all that apply.)
   A. Aneurysm
   B. Dissection
   C. Intramural hematoma
   D. Penetrating aortic ulcer

2. What is the most likely cause of this patient's
   abnormality?
   A. Marfan syndrome
   B. Dissection
   C. Intramural hematoma
   D. Penetrating aortic ulcer

3. What is the cause of a penetrating aortic ulcer?
   A. Infection
   B. Trauma
   C. Iatrogenic
   D. Atherosclerosis

4. What is the most appropriate management?
   A. No treatment
   B. Antihypertensive medication
   C. Anticoagulation
   D. Surgery

Pseudoaneurysm Secondary to Penetrating Aortic Ulcer

1. B, C, and D

2. D

3. D

4. D

Reference

Reddy GP, Gunn M, Mitsumori LM, et al: Multislice CT and MRI of the thoracic aorta. In Webb WR, Higgins CB, editors: *Thoracic imaging: pulmonary and cardiovascular radiology*, ed 2, Philadelphia, 2010, Lippincott Williams & Wilkin.

Cross-Reference

Cardiac Imaging: The REQUISITES, ed 3, pp 377–379.

Comment

Etiology, Pathology, and Management

An aortic pseudoaneurysm can be due to a penetrating atherosclerotic ulcer, infection, trauma (deceleration injury—although this is an unusual location), or iatrogenic injury. Pseudoaneurysms are characterized by disruption of one or more layers of the vessel wall, whereas true aneurysms have intact walls. Because pseudoaneurysms are characterized by disruption of one or more layers of the arterial wall, they are at risk for rupture, and management usually involves surgical resection.

Imaging

CT and MRI can be used to establish the diagnosis of a thoracic aortic aneurysm. Disruption of the wall is difficult to identify by imaging examination. If the outpouching has a relatively narrow ostium (<50% of the aneurysm diameter), it is likely a pseudoaneurysm (Figs. A and B), whereas an aneurysm with a wide ostium is likely to be a true aneurysm.

Acute Aortic Syndrome

There are three diseases that are classically considered to be a part of the acute aortic syndrome: aortic dissection, intramural hematoma, and penetrating aortic ulcer. Some authors propose including three additional entities: aortitis, intimal tear from trauma, and intraluminal aortic thrombus. Acute aortic syndrome diseases are classified under the Stanford system. Stanford type A lesions involve the ascending aorta and generally are treated surgically or endovascularly with stent grafts. Stanford type B lesions do not involve the ascending aorta and generally are managed medically unless complications develop.

Notes

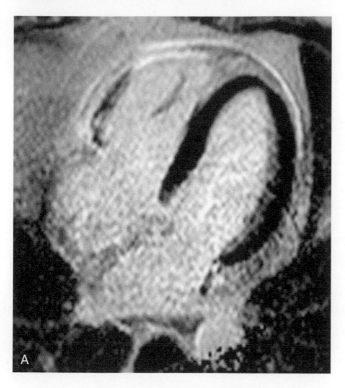

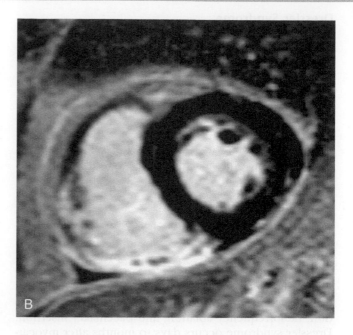

History: No patient history is available.

1. Which should be included in the differential diagnosis for pericardial thickening? (Choose all that apply.)
   A. Acute pericarditis
   B. Constrictive pericarditis
   C. Chronic pericarditis
   D. Pericardial metastasis
   E. Congestive heart failure

2. What sequence and imaging plane are shown in Fig. A?
   A. Inversion recovery late gadolinium enhancement MRI, short-axis view
   B. Inversion recovery late gadolinium enhancement MRI, four-chamber view
   C. Cine steady-state free precession (SSFP), short-axis view
   D. Cine SSFP, four-chamber view

3. Which of the following is a postcardiac injury syndrome?
   A. Dressler syndrome
   B. Acute coronary syndrome
   C. Broken heart syndrome
   D. Hypoplastic left heart syndrome

4. What would be the most likely presentation for this patient?
   A. A 45-year-old man presents with intractable ascites and lower extremity edema. He underwent high-dose mantle radiation therapy for Hodgkin lymphoma as a child. Cardiac angiography shows equalization of ventricular pressures.
   B. A 45-year-old man presents with severe substernal chest pain not relieved with nitroglycerin. There is ST segment elevation in the inferior ECG leads.
   C. A 45-year-old man presents 3 weeks after myocardial infarction with pleuritic chest pain, fever, and dyspnea.
   D. A 45-year-old man presents with progressive dyspnea on exertion following a recent divorce. Echocardiography shows apical ballooning and reduced ejection fraction.

Dressler Syndrome

1. A, B, C, and D

2. B

3. A

4. C

Reference

Wessman DE, Stafford CM: The postcardiac injury syndrome: case report and review of the literature, *South Med J* 99(3):309-314, 2006.

Cross-Reference

Cardiac Imaging: The REQUISITES, ed 3, pp 267, 272.

Comment

Epidemiology

Postcardiac injury syndromes can be seen after myocardial infarction, cardiac surgery, percutaneous intervention, radiofrequency ablation, and pacemaker insertion. Dressler syndrome occurs days to months after myocardial infarction and is thought to be an autoantibody response to normal cardiac tissue exposed after the insult. At the present time, Dressler syndrome occurs in less than 1% of patients after myocardial infarction. This decreased incidence is thought to be due to earlier reperfusion and the antiinflammatory effects of cardiac drugs given after myocardial infarction.

Imaging Findings and Treatment

Advanced imaging is infrequently performed to diagnose this condition. The most common finding is pericardial thickening with enhancement (Figs. A and B). Additional findings associated with Dressler syndrome include exudative pericardial and pleural effusions. The prognosis is good because patients respond favorably to nonsteroidal antiinflammatory drugs (NSAIDs) and corticosteroids. Feared complications of postcardiac injury syndromes are graft occlusion after coronary artery bypass graft surgery and hemorrhagic cardiac tamponade in the setting of anticoagulation therapy. One small study showed that NSAIDs, corticosteroids, and aspirin reduced the risk of graft occlusion from 86% to 16%.

Notes

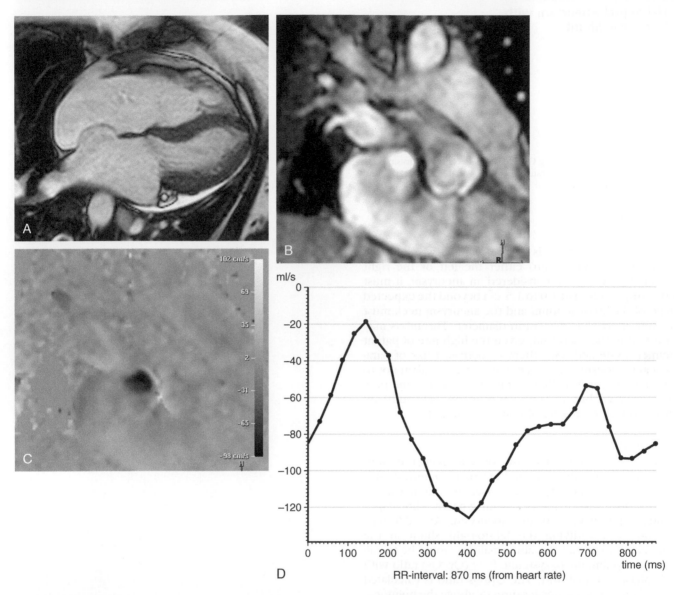

History: A 51-year-old woman presents with palpitations and a severely enlarged right ventricle on transthoracic echocardiogram.

1. What should be included in the differential diagnosis for a left-to-right shunt? (Choose all that apply.)
   A. Atrial septal defect (ASD)
   B. Partial anomalous pulmonary venous return (PAPVR)
   C. Ventricular septal defect (VSD)
   D. Patent ductus arteriosus (PDA)
   E. Meandering pulmonary vein

2. What imaging sequence is shown in Figs. B and C?
   A. Steady-state free precession (SSFP)
   B. Velocity-encoded cine (VEC) phase contrast
   C. Double inversion recovery
   D. Late gadolinium enhancement

3. What is the most debilitating complication of this entity?
   A. Paradoxical embolism with stroke
   B. Mitral regurgitation
   C. Malignant degeneration
   D. Peripheral limb ischemia

4. What is the most likely diagnosis?
   A. Cardiac mass
   B. Mitral stenosis
   C. VSD
   D. Atrial septal aneurysm

CASE 64

Atrial Septal Aneurysm with Intracardiac Shunt

1. A, B, C, and D

2. B

3. A

4. D

Reference

Dodd JD, Aquino SL, Holmvang G, et al: Cardiac septal aneurysm mimicking pseudomass: appearance on ECG-gated cardiac MRI and MDCT, *AJR Am J Roentgenol* 188(6):W550–W553, 2007.

Comment

Diagnosis

Atrial septal aneurysm is uncommon; it is a discrete bulge of the septum into either the left or the right atrium (Fig. A). To be considered an aneurysm, it must protrude greater than 1.0 to 1.5 cm beyond the expected plane of the atrial septum, and the aneurysm neck must measure more than 1.5 cm in diameter. Thrombus may form within the aneurysm; given the high rate of patent foramen ovale and ASD, there is increased risk of paradoxical embolism and stroke. Care must be taken not to confuse this entity with a cardiac mass on routine nongated chest CT because there may be unopacified blood owing to lack of mixing of contrast material.

Cardiac MRI

Cardiac MRI has the added value of quantifying the shunt fraction through the use of VEC phase contrast MRI (Figs. B-D). As shown in this case, the shunt can be directly quantified with phase imaging by choosing a plane perpendicular to the aneurysm. An additional method of quantifying the left-to-right shunt in the absence of other valvular abnormalities would be to calculate the pulmonic-to-systemic flow (Qp/Qs) ratio with VEC phase contrast MRI. The Qp/Qs ratio is calculated by performing phase images directly above the pulmonic and aortic valves. In normal patients, the blood leaving the left and right ventricles should be roughly equal. In patients with a shunt, the Qp/Qs ratio does not equal 1 and is directly related to the shunted fraction.

Notes

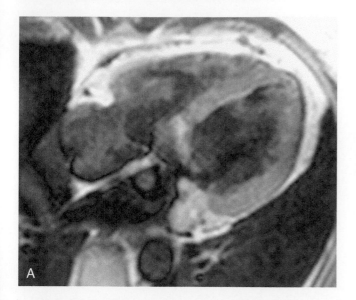

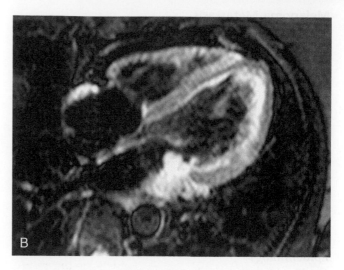

History: A patient presents with arrhythmia.

1. What should be included in the differential diagnosis for a T1 hyperintense cardiac mass on a non–contrast-enhanced image? (Choose all that apply.)
   A. Lipoma
   B. Lipomatous hypertrophy of the interatrial septum
   C. Lung cancer metastasis
   D. Myxoma
   E. Melanoma metastasis

2. What is the most useful way to differentiate a fat-containing lesion from a melanin-containing lesion?
   A. Contrast-enhanced T1-weighted images
   B. Fat-suppressed T1-weighted images
   C. Cine steady-state free precession
   D. Velocity-encoded cine phase contrast

3. What is the most common cardiac tumor?
   A. Lipoma
   B. Angiosarcoma
   C. Myxoma
   D. Metastasis

4. What is the most common patient presentation for this entity?
   A. Arrhythmia
   B. Asymptomatic
   C. Chest pain
   D. Pneumothorax

Melanoma Metastasis

1. A, B, and E

2. B

3. D

4. B

Reference

Tesolin M, Lapierre C, Oligny L, et al: Cardiac metastases from melanoma, *Radiographics* 25(1):249-253, 2005.

Cross-Reference

Cardiac Imaging: The REQUISITES, ed 3, pp 277-278.

Comment

Epidemiology

Cardiac metastasis is the most common cardiac tumor. The most frequent metastases are from lung or breast cancer. However, melanoma is more likely to metastasize to the heart; more than 50% of patients with known melanoma have evidence of metastatic disease at autopsy. Melanoma metastases are difficult to diagnose because they are commonly asymptomatic. Most patients who are symptomatic present with arrhythmia.

Differential Diagnosis and Treatment

Melanoma metastases are characteristically hyperintense on T1-weighted images because of the presence of melanin. They are T2 hyperintense and enhance with contrast agent administration, which are important features to differentiate from thrombus. MRI is the test of choice in patients with suspected metastatic disease. Surgery may be performed in select cases to treat an isolated melanoma metastasis.

Imaging

Axial T1-weighted black blood imaging (Fig. A) shows a mildly hyperintense, irregularly shaped mass within the lateral left atrial wall. The mass remains hyperintense on fat-suppressed T2-weighted black blood imaging (Fig. B).

Notes

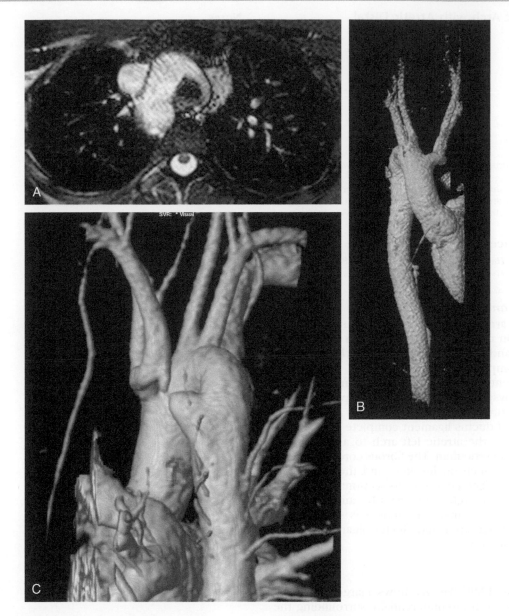

History: No patient history is available.

1. Which of the following entities are considered vascular rings or slings? (Choose all that apply.)
   A. Left aortic arch with aberrant right subclavian artery
   B. Right aortic arch with aberrant left subclavian artery
   C. Right aortic arch with mirror image branching
   D. Anomalous left pulmonary artery
   E. Double aortic arch

2. What is the anomaly in this case?
   A. Pulmonary sling
   B. Right arch with mirror image branching
   C. Right arch with aberrant left subclavian artery
   D. Double aortic arch

3. What is the most likely clinical presentation in this adult patient?
   A. Asymptomatic
   B. Wheezing and dyspnea
   C. Hemoptysis
   D. Dysphagia

4. What is the most common symptomatic vascular ring?
   A. Double aortic arch
   B. Right aortic arch with aberrant left subclavian artery
   C. Left aortic arch with aberrant right subclavian artery
   D. Right aortic arch with mirror image branching

CASE 66

Double Aortic Arch with Atretic Distal Left Arch

1. B, D, and E

2. D

3. B

4. A

References

Kellenberger CJ: Aortic arch malformations, *Pediatr Radiol* 40(6):876–884, 2010.

Schlesinger AE, Krishnamurthy R, Sena LM, et al: Incomplete double aortic arch with atresia of the distal left arch: distinctive imaging appearance, *AJR Am J Roentgenol* 184(5):1634–1639, 2005.

Cross-Reference

Cardiac Imaging: The REQUISITES, ed 3, pp 414–418.

Comment

Epidemiology and Management

Double aortic arch is the most common symptomatic vascular ring. In most cases, the right arch is dominant being higher and larger than the left arch. A double aortic arch compresses and narrows the trachea and esophagus, eventually leading to tracheomalacia with symptoms of dyspnea, wheezing, and dysphagia. Infrequently, a portion of the left arch is atretic. A nonpatent fibrous cord and ductus ligament complete the vascular ring by tethering the atretic left arch to a descending thoracic aortic diverticulum. The fibrous cord and ductus ligament are not seen on imaging, and their positions must be inferred. The goal of cross-sectional imaging is to determine which arch is dominant because this influences surgical management. Treatment is surgical ligation of the smaller arch and ductus ligament via an ipsilateral thoracotomy.

Imaging

Axial T2-weighted MRI (Fig. A) shows a larger right arch and smaller left arch circumferentially surrounding the upper trachea anteriorly and esophagus posteriorly. Three-dimensional volume-rendered magnetic resonance angiography (MRA) (Fig. B) of the aorta confirms a double aortic arch with the right arch being higher and larger than the left arch. Posterior volume-rendered imaging (Fig. C) shows that the left arch is incomplete and atretic distally at the junction with a descending thoracic aortic diverticulum.

Differential Diagnosis

Differentiation of incomplete double aortic arch with atretic left arch from right aortic arch with mirror image branching is difficult. Imaging clues that favor the former diagnosis include a symmetric appearance of bilateral common carotid and subclavian arteries originating from the right arch and atretic left arch and a diverticulum of the descending thoracic aorta (both present in this case).

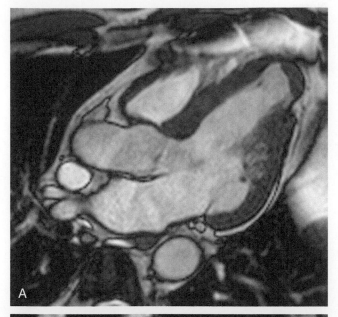

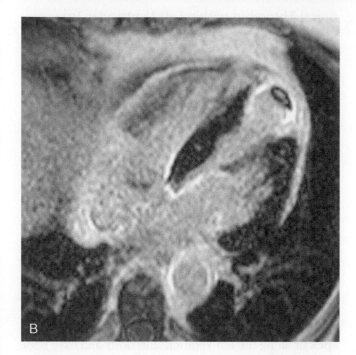

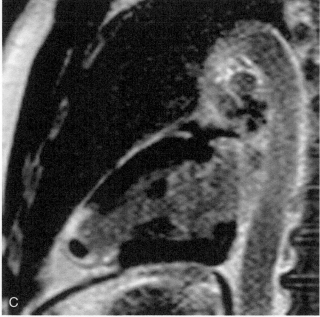

History: A patient has a cardiac mass identified on echocardiography.

1. What should be included in the differential diagnosis for Figs. A-C? (Choose all that apply.)
   A. Sarcoidosis
   B. Left ventricle infarction with microvascular obstruction
   C. Amyloidosis
   D. Left ventricle infarction with thrombus

2. What is the major finding?
   A. True aneurysm
   B. Tumor
   C. Acute infarction
   D. Myocarditis

3. What is the best imaging clue or test to distinguish a true ventricular aneurysm from a false ventricular aneurysm?
   A. Biopsy
   B. Location
   C. Thrombus
   D. Size of neck

4. How is a true aneurysm treated if the patient has refractory arrhythmia?
   A. No treatment
   B. Surgical resection of aneurysm
   C. Ethanol ablation
   D. Multidrug therapy

CASE 67

Apical Thrombus within Left Ventricular True Aneurysm after Myocardial Infarction

1. B and D

2. A

3. D

4. B

Reference

Kumbasar B, Wu KC, Kamel IR, et al: Left ventricular true aneurysm: diagnosis of myocardial viability shown on MR imaging, *AJR Am J Roentgenol* 179(2):472-474, 2002.

Cross-Reference

Cardiac Imaging: The REQUISITES, ed 3, pp 235-237

Comment

Aneurysm Type

Two types of ventricular aneurysm can occur after myocardial infarction—true and false aneurysms. True aneurysms are commonly located at the left ventricular apex or along the left ventricle anteriorly and have wide necks. False aneurysms, or pseudoaneurysms, are commonly located along the left ventricle inferiorly and posteriorly and have narrow necks. Pseudoaneurysms are contained only by pericardium, whereas true aneurysms are contained by infarcted myocardium and pericardium. Distinguishing between these two types of aneurysm is important because treatments differ. True aneurysms have a low likelihood of complications and are generally treated conservatively. False aneurysms have a high rate of rupture and are managed surgically.

Imaging

Cine steady-state free precession (SSFP) left ventricular outflow tract view shows a focal outpouching of the left ventricular apex with a wide neck and thinned myocardium (Fig. A). Late gadolinium enhancement four-chamber and vertical long-axis images show circumferential enhancement corresponding to the region of outpouching at the left ventricular apex (Figs. B and C). The adjacent myocardium is of normal thickness and does not enhance. There is an oval-shaped nonenhancing lesion, consistent with thrombus.

Differential Diagnosis

In addition to the location and size of the neck of the aneurysm, late gadolinium enhancement imaging may be useful in differentiating between aneurysm types. As in this case, a true aneurysm is contained by infarcted myocardium and is readily identified by transmural late gadolinium enhancement (Figs. B and C). A false aneurysm has no residual myocardium because it represents a contained ventricular rupture, and its wall does not exhibit late gadolinium enhancement.

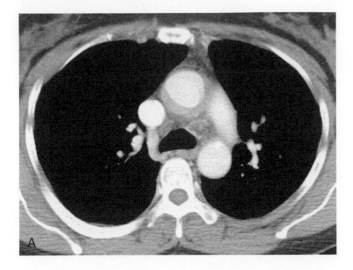

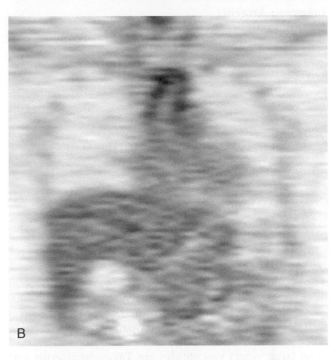

History: A 35-year-old woman presents with fatigue, weight loss, arm claudication, and elevated erythrocyte sedimentation rate.

1. What should be included in the differential diagnosis for fluorodeoxyglucose (FDG) uptake shown in Fig. B? (Choose all that apply.)
   A. Atherosclerosis
   B. Takayasu arteritis
   C. Giant cell arteritis
   D. Intramural hematoma

2. What is the imaging finding seen in Fig. A?
   A. Atherosclerosis
   B. Aortic wall thickening
   C. Sternal fracture
   D. Intimal flap

3. What is the most likely diagnosis in this 35-year-old woman presenting with arm claudication and an elevated sedimentation rate?
   A. Atherosclerosis
   B. Giant cell arteritis
   C. Takayasu arteritis
   D. Aortic dissection

4. What is the role of PET in this disease?
   A. Monitor response to therapy
   B. No role
   C. Guide surgical therapy
   D. Differentiate this disease from atherosclerosis

Takayasu Arteritis

1. A, B, C, and D

2. B

3. C

4. A

Reference

James OG, Christensen JD, Wong TZ, et al: Utility of FDG PET/CT in inflammatory cardiovascular disease, *Radiographics* 31(5):1271–1286, 2011.

Cross-Reference

Cardiac Imaging: The REQUISITES, ed 3, pp 393–394.

Comment

Differential Diagnosis

Axial contrast-enhanced CT shows ascending aortic wall thickening with enhancement (Fig. A). Coronal PET shows increased FDG activity in the ascending aortic wall (Fig. B). The main differential diagnoses include atherosclerosis and a large vessel vasculitis. The two main large vessel vasculitides are Takayasu arteritis and giant cell arteritis. Takayasu arteritis most commonly affects females 10 to 40 years old, whereas giant cell arteritis occurs in patients older than 50 years.

Monitoring Response to Therapy

The role of PET in diagnosing and monitoring treatment response in patients with an inflammatory arteritis is evolving. Often PET may be the first study to suggest a vasculitis when it is performed in patients referred for fever of unknown origin or nonspecific constitutional symptoms. The characteristic finding of a large vessel vasculitis is circumferential increased FDG activity within the involved vessel wall (Fig. B). This increased FDG activity represents active disease and is relatively sensitive and specific for the diagnosis in the presence of elevated inflammatory markers. PET is also useful in monitoring disease response to antiinflammatory medications. PET shows treatment response earlier than anatomic imaging. Decreased vessel wall metabolic activity correlates with symptom resolution and reduced inflammatory blood markers.

Notes

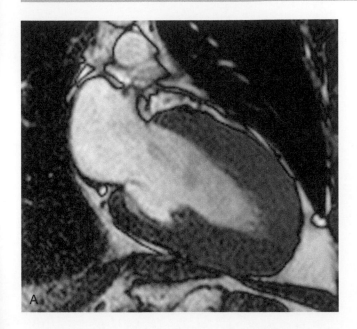

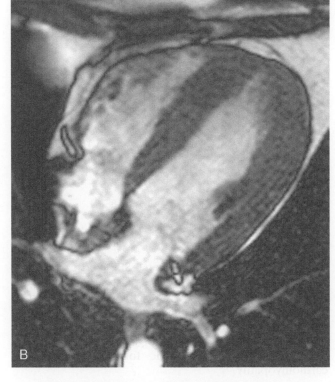

History: A patient experiences sudden cardiac death.

1. What should be included in the differential diagnosis? (Choose all that apply.)
   A. Systemic hypertension
   B. Aortic stenosis
   C. Amyloidosis
   D. Aortic regurgitation
   E. Hypertrophic cardiomyopathy

2. What is the main imaging finding?
   A. Ventricular chamber dilation
   B. Concentric left ventricular hypertrophy
   C. Fatty infiltration of the right ventricular free wall
   D. Asymmetric septal hypertrophy

3. What is the most likely diagnosis in a 20-year-old man with sudden cardiac death and no significant past medical history?
   A. Arrhythmogenic right ventricular dysplasia
   B. Anomalous left coronary artery from the pulmonary artery
   C. Obstructing left atrial myxoma
   D. Hypertrophic cardiomyopathy

4. What is the mode of inheritance for this condition?
   A. Sporadic occurrence
   B. Autosomal recessive
   C. Autosomal dominant
   D. X-linked

Concentric Hypertrophic Cardiomyopathy

1. A, B, C, and E

2. B

3. D

4. C

Reference

Chun EJ, Choi SI, Jin KN, et al: Hypertrophic cardiomyopathy: assessment with MR imaging and multidetector CT, *Radiographics* 30(5):1309-1328, 2010.

Cross-Reference

Cardiac Imaging: The REQUISITES, ed 3, pp 88–91.

Comment

Imaging

Cine steady-state free precession (SSFP) vertical long-axis and four-chamber views at end-diastole show circumferential left ventricular wall thickening measuring greater than 15 mm in diameter (Figs. A and B). This patient had no systemic condition to explain this degree of wall thickening. The findings are consistent with the concentric or symmetric form of hypertrophic cardiomyopathy.

Criteria for Diagnosis

The maximal left ventricular wall thickness must measure 15 mm or greater in end-diastole to suggest a diagnosis of hypertrophic cardiomyopathy (Figs. A and B). Also, there must be no systemic condition (e.g., hypertension or aortic stenosis) to explain the degree of left ventricular thickening.

Differential Diagnosis

Concentric hypertrophic cardiomyopathy is a less common form of hypertrophic cardiomyopathy. This entity can be diagnosed only after exclusion of other causes of concentric left ventricular wall thickening (e.g., amyloidosis, sarcoidosis, athletic heart, systemic hypertension, and aortic stenosis). MRI is ideally suited to differentiate among the various causes of symmetric left ventricular wall thickening through the use of late gadolinium enhancement and T2-weighted imaging. Amyloidosis is a restrictive cardiomyopathy and characteristically has diffuse subendocardial late gadolinium enhancement. Sarcoidosis causes patchy increased T2 signal and late gadolinium enhancement within portions of the myocardium. Late gadolinium enhancement in sarcoidosis and amyloidosis does not correspond to a vascular territory. Left ventricular wall thickness rarely exceeds 15 mm in patients with aortic stenosis and systemic hypertension, and there is usually no late gadolinium enhancement.

Notes

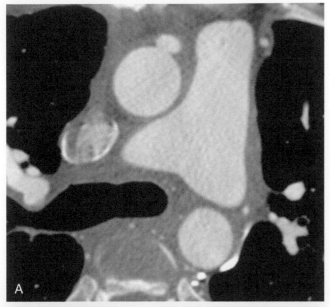

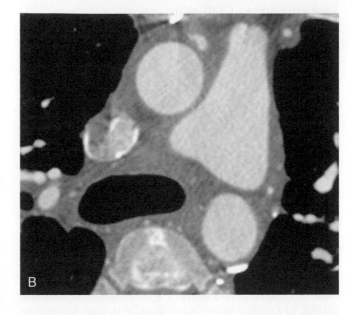

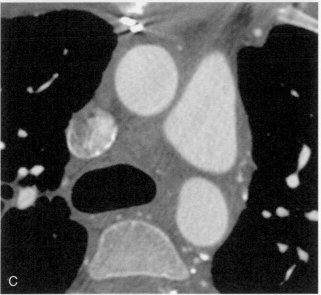

History: A patient presents with recurrent chest pain less than 1 month after undergoing coronary artery bypass graft (CABG) surgery

1. What should be included in the differential diagnosis for this patient history? (Choose all that apply.)
   A. Graft occlusion
   B. Sternal infection
   C. Pneumonia
   D. Pulmonary embolism
   E. Pericardial effusion

2. What imaging finding is shown in Figs. A-C?
   A. Pulmonary embolism
   B. Superior vena cava thrombus
   C. Saphenous vein graft occlusion
   D. Aortic dissection

3. Which of the following vascular conduits is the most robust for use in CABG surgery?
   A. Left internal mammary artery (LIMA)
   B. Saphenous vein
   C. Radial artery
   D. Gastroepiploic artery

4. What is a major advantage of a saphenous vein graft over the LIMA graft?
   A. Improved cardiac event-free survival
   B. Conduit length
   C. High long-term patency
   D. Decreased postoperative mortality

Saphenous Vein Graft with Complete Occlusion

1. A, B, C, D, and E

2. C

3. A

4. B

Reference

Frazier AA, Qureshi F, Read KM, et al: Coronary artery bypass grafts: assessment with multidetector CT in the early and late postoperative settings, *Radiographics* 25(4):881–896, 2005.

Cross-Reference

Cardiac Imaging: The REQUISITES, ed 3, pp 229–231.

Comment

Imaging

Figs. A-C from a coronary CT angiogram (extending caudal to cranial) show a proximally patent saphenous vein graft arising from the anterior ascending aorta. Fig. C shows near-complete occlusion of the graft.

Complications of CABG

CT angiography is useful in the evaluation of symptomatic patients after CABG surgery. CT angiography is able to diagnose accurately both early and late complications of surgery. Early complications (<1 month after surgery) include saphenous vein graft thrombosis, sternal infection, pericardial or pleural effusion, and pulmonary embolism. Late complications (>1 month after surgery) include graft stenosis or occlusion or graft aneurysm. CT angiography is also useful in preoperative planning before repeat CABG surgery. The main goal of imaging in these patients is to depict the course of the LIMA and saphenous vein graft with respect to the sternum to avoid injury with repeat sternotomy.

Notes

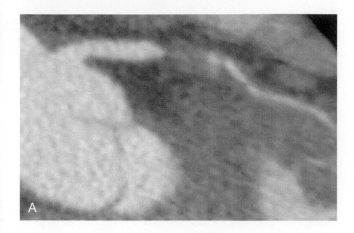

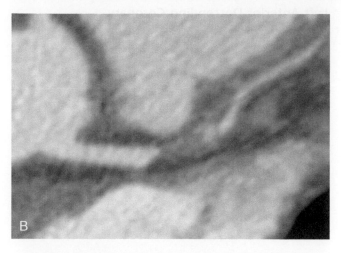

History: No patient history is available.

1. In which patients is CT angiography of the coronary arteries indicated? (Choose all that apply.)
   A. Patients with low pretest probability presenting with chest pain
   B. Patients with intermediate pretest probability presenting with chest pain
   C. Patients with high pretest probability with typical signs and symptoms of coronary artery disease (CAD)
   D. Asymptomatic patients
   E. Patients with chest pain and chest radiograph showing a pneumothorax

2. What percentage of patients presenting to the emergency department with chest pain are determined to have a coronary event at the time of discharge?
   A. 5%
   B. 25%
   C. 50%
   D. 80%

3. What reduces the specificity of CT angiography in accurately depicting the degree of coronary artery stenosis?
   A. Coronary calcium score greater than 400
   B. Low heart rate
   C. Extensive noncalcified plaque
   D. Thin body habitus

4. What is the recommendation for this patient?
   A. Coronary stent
   B. Medical management
   C. Coronary artery bypass graft surgery
   D. Coronary angiography

Left Anterior Descending Coronary Artery Occlusion

1. A and B

2. B

3. A

4. D

Reference

Zimmet JM, Miller JM: Coronary artery CTA: imaging of atherosclerosis in the coronary arteries and reporting of coronary artery CTA findings, *Tech Vasc Interv Radiol* 9(4):218–226, 2006.

Cross-Reference

Cardiac Imaging: The REQUISITES, ed 3, pp 248–261.

Comment

Imaging

Two multiplanar reformatted images from CT angiography show complete occlusion of the left anterior descending (LAD) coronary artery by noncalcified plaque (Figs. A and B). The distal LAD is diminutive. LAD occlusion was confirmed via cardiac catheterization with distal reconstitution of the LAD via collaterals. Percutaneous stent placement was performed after determining the presence of residual myocardial viability with delayed thallium imaging.

Management

Coronary angiography remains the gold standard to assess coronary anatomy and to determine the degree of vessel narrowing. The main limitation of the test is that it is an invasive procedure with potential serious complications. CT angiography is useful in the evaluation of patients with a low or intermediate pretest probability of disease. A negative test essentially rules out significant pathology. The patient is able to be discharged earlier, and there is evidence of significant cost savings. A positive test must be confirmed with invasive coronary angiography. In this case, the patient has a positive CT angiogram with complete LAD occlusion and requires confirmation and potentially treatment with coronary angiography.

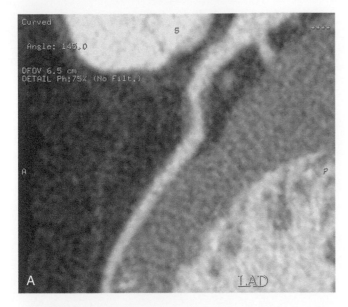

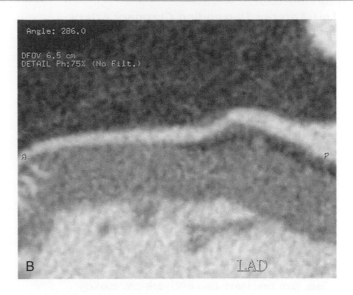

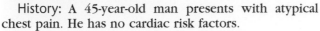

History: A 45-year-old man presents with atypical chest pain. He has no cardiac risk factors.

1. What should be included in the differential diagnosis? (Choose all that apply.)
   A. Coronary artery dissection
   B. Thrombus
   C. Atherosclerosis
   D. Aneurysm

2. What is a major advantage of CT angiography over nuclear medicine scintigraphic evaluation of chest pain?
   A. Diagnosis of other diseases
   B. Physiologic information
   C. Functional information
   D. Ability to evaluate sedentary patients

3. In addition to coronary artery stenosis involving the LAD coronary artery, what is the additional finding?
   A. Myocardial bridge
   B. Thrombus
   C. Coronary aneurysm
   D. Positive remodeling

4. What is the recommendation for this patient?
   A. Coronary stent
   B. Medical management
   C. Coronary artery bypass graft surgery
   D. Coronary angiography

Left Anterior Descending Coronary Artery Stenosis (<50%) with Positive Remodeling

1. C

2. A

3. D

4. B

References

Kröner ES, van Velzen JE, Boogers MJ, et al: Positive remodeling on coronary computed tomography as a marker for plaque vulnerability on virtual histology intravascular ultrasound, *Am J Cardiol* 107(12): 1725-1729, 2011.

Schoenhagen P, Ziada KM, Vince DG, et al: Arterial remodeling and coronary artery disease: the concept of "dilated" versus "obstructive" coronary atherosclerosis, *J Am Coll Cardiol* 38(2):297-306, 2001.

Zimmet JM, Miller JM: Coronary artery CTA: imaging of atherosclerosis in the coronary arteries and reporting of coronary artery CTA findings, *Tech Vasc Interv Radiol* 9(4):218-226, 2006.

Cross-Reference

Cardiac Imaging: The REQUISITES, ed 3, pp 248-261.

Comment

Imaging

Multiplanar reformatted images from CT angiography show focal stenosis (<50%) of the LAD coronary artery by noncalcified plaque (Figs. A and B). The vessel is expanded outward in the region of atherosclerosis, which is known as positive remodeling.

Prognosis

The traditional thinking regarding coronary atherosclerosis is that it leads to progressive vessel narrowing as plaque is deposited within the intima; this is known as negative remodeling. However, certain plaque does not initially cause vessel narrowing but instead expands the media and external elastic membrane. This expansion causes the vessel to bulge outward in the region of atherosclerosis as a protective mechanism to limit the degree of luminal narrowing (Figs. A and B). This phenomenon is known as positive remodeling. In this process, the luminal cross-sectional area is not affected until the plaque causes a 40% area reduction. Catheter angiography is unable to detect the process of positive remodeling, whereas CT angiography can depict not only the lumen but also the outer wall. The process of positive remodeling is associated with vulnerable plaque owing to a larger lipid core and macrophage count; this helps explain why plaque rupture often occurs at sites of only minimal or modest stenosis. Negative remodeling is often associated with stable coronary syndromes. In the future, CT angiography may be used to identify positive remodeling because it is a marker of plaque vulnerability.

Notes

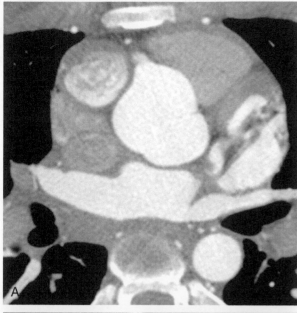

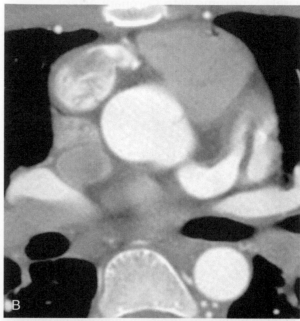

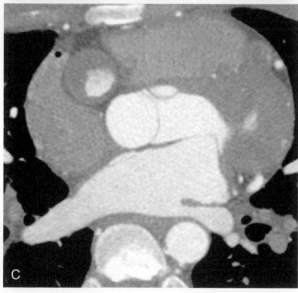

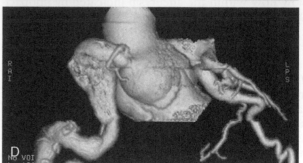

History: A 19-year-old Japanese man has a history of a severe childhood illness.

1. What are potential causes of coronary artery aneurysm? (Choose all that apply.)
   A. Takayasu arteritis
   B. Iatrogenic
   C. Atherosclerosis
   D. Infection
   E. Anomalous left coronary artery from the pulmonary artery (ALCAPA)

2. What is the most likely diagnosis if the coronary artery abnormalities have been present since an early childhood illness?
   A. Iatrogenic injury
   B. Atherosclerosis
   C. Kawasaki disease
   D. Mycotic aneurysm

3. Which of the following is currently used to prevent this complication in Kawasaki disease?
   A. Vaccination
   B. γ-Globulin
   C. Stent placement
   D. Beta blocker

4. What is the most likely patient presentation for a coronary artery aneurysm?
   A. Rupture
   B. Thrombosis
   C. Distal embolization
   D. Asymptomatic

CASE 73

Kawasaki Syndrome with Coronary Artery Aneurysms

1. A, B, C, and D

2. C

3. B

4. D

Reference

Díaz-Zamudio M, Bacilio-Pérez U, Herrera-Zarza MC, et al: Coronary artery aneurysms and ectasia: role of coronary CT angiography, *Radiographics* 29(7):1939-1954, 2009.

Cross-Reference

Cardiac Imaging: The REQUISITES, ed 3, pp 220-223.

Comment

Imaging

Multiple axial images of the coronary arteries show a large right coronary artery aneurysm (Figs. A-C). There is slow flow within the aneurysm indicated by unopacified blood (Figs. A-C). There is also an aneurysm of the left main coronary artery (Fig. B). This patient had a previous history of Kawasaki syndrome.

Definition of Aneurysm or Ectasia

Coronary artery dilation can be classified as either vessel ectasia or an aneurysm. Vascular ectasia refers to diffuse dilation of a coronary artery. Ectasia often occurs in vessels with a high-flow state owing to a coronary artery fistula, coronary anomaly, or opposite vessel coronary artery stenosis. A coronary artery aneurysm is defined by a dilated segment that is 1.5 times larger than an adjacent normal segment and does not exceed 50% of the total vessel length. In children younger than 5 years, a coronary artery is considered aneurysmal when it exceeds 4 mm in diameter.

Classification

Coronary artery aneurysms are further classified into true or false aneurysms. True aneurysm walls are composed of all three vessel layers—the intima, media, and adventitia. Conversely, false aneurysms are contained by only one or two vessel layers and are more prone to rupture. False aneurysms are typically the sequela of iatrogenic injury during cardiac catheterization or blunt trauma.

Demographics

In the United States, coronary artery aneurysms are most commonly seen in association with atherosclerosis. In Japan, Kawasaki syndrome is the most common cause of coronary aneurysms. Kawasaki syndrome is a self-limited panarteritis that affects multiple organ systems. It may be secondary to an infectious process or an autoimmune reaction. The feared complications of Kawasaki syndrome are related to the cardiovascular system and include coronary artery aneurysms, premature atherosclerosis, and myocardial infarction. Approximately 25%

of untreated patients may develop coronary artery aneurysms with complications often occurring years after the initial diagnosis. Prompt recognition of this syndrome allows clinicians to initiate early γ-globulin and aspirin therapy, which reduces the risk of developing a coronary artery aneurysm to 5%.

Notes

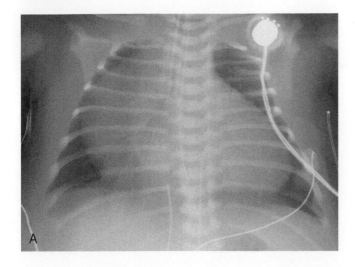

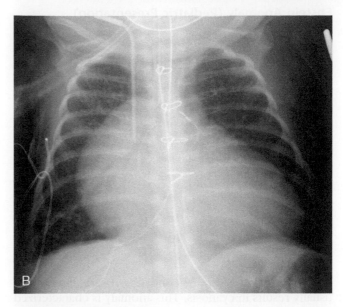

History: Two infants present with the same type of congenital heart disease. Patient 2 is status post surgical correction.

1. What should be included in the differential diagnosis? (Choose all that apply.)
   A. Transposition of great arteries
   B. Ebstein anomaly
   C. Pulmonary atresia with restrictive ventricular septal defect
   D. Tetralogy of Fallot
   E. Atrial septal defect

2. What is the most likely diagnosis?
   A. Hypoplastic left heart syndrome
   B. Transposition of great arteries
   C. Tetralogy of Fallot
   D. Ebstein anomaly

3. What is the usual clinical presentation of this condition in neonates (<2 months old)?
   A. Cyanosis
   B. Incidental heart murmur
   C. Heart failure with poor feeding and failure to thrive
   D. Brain abscess

4. Maternal ingestion of which drug during pregnancy is most commonly associated with Ebstein anomaly?
   A. Atorvastatin
   B. Lithium
   C. Atenolol
   D. Warfarin

CASE 74

Ebstein Anomaly (Pediatric Presentation)

1. B and C

2. D

3. A

4. B

Reference

Ferguson EC, Krishnamurthy R, Oldham SA: Classic imaging signs of congenital cardiovascular abnormalities, *Radiographics* 27(5):1323–1334, 2007.

Cross-Reference

Cardiac Imaging: The REQUISITES, ed 3, pp 206–207.

Comment

Overview

Ebstein anomaly is a rare congenital heart disease that usually results in cyanosis. This anomaly is characterized by ventricular displacement of the tricuspid valve leaflets resulting in a common ventriculoatrial chamber and often severe tricuspid regurgitation. Over time, there is progressive dilation of all right-sided chambers, which leads to increased tricuspid regurgitation and further chamber dilation. Most patients with Ebstein anomaly also have an atrial septal defect or patent foramen ovale. As right-sided pressures increase, a right-to-left shunt develops leading to cyanosis. This entity is characterized by normal to decreased pulmonary vasculature and massive right atrial enlargement, which may fill the entire right hemithorax. The aorta and pulmonary artery are typically small, leading to the characteristic box-shaped heart (Figs. A and B).

Associations

Ebstein anomaly is associated with an atrial septal defect or patent foramen ovale in approximately 90% of patients. Less common associations include supraventricular tachycardia (25% to 50%), pulmonary atresia or stenosis (25%), and Wolff-Parkinson-White syndrome (10%).

Imaging

A frontal radiograph shows massive cardiac enlargement (so-called wall-to-wall heart) and decreased pulmonary vasculature (Fig. A). Ebstein anomaly is the major consideration in a cyanotic patient. Much less common causes of this radiographic appearance include severe pulmonic stenosis with restrictive atrial septal defect, tricuspid atresia with a restrictive atrial septal defect, and pulmonary atresia with a restrictive ventricular septal defect.

Notes

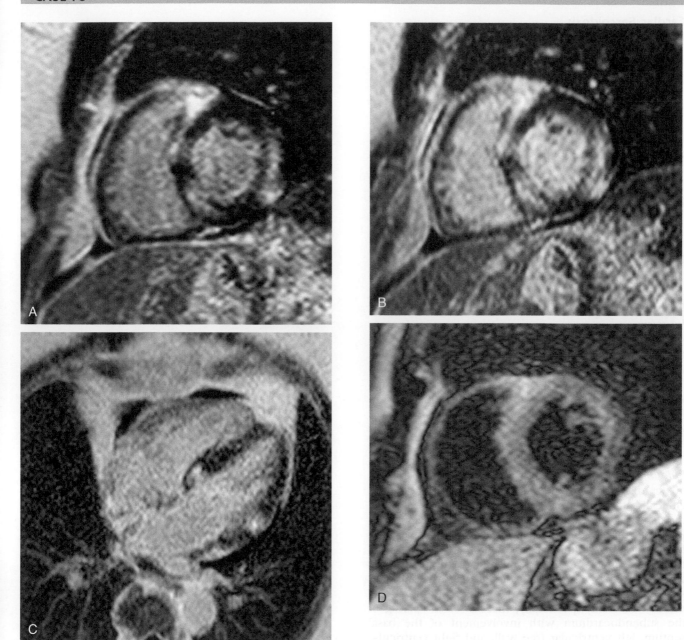

History: A 44-year-old woman presents with cardiac arrhythmia.

1. What should be included in the differential diagnosis? (Choose all that apply.)
   A. Myocarditis
   B. Infarction
   C. Ischemia
   D. Athlete's heart
   E. Sarcoidosis

2. What is the likely diagnosis if this patient had long-standing bilateral hilar lymphadenopathy?
   A. Myocarditis
   B. Infarction
   C. Athlete's heart
   D. Sarcoidosis

3. Which organ or system is most commonly affected by sarcoidosis?
   A. Lungs and lymph nodes
   B. Heart
   C. Liver
   D. Central nervous system

4. What type of cardiomyopathy is most commonly associated with sarcoidosis?
   A. Dilated
   B. Restrictive
   C. Hypertrophic
   D. Noncompaction

CASE 75

Cardiac Sarcoidosis

1. A and E

2. D

3. A

4. B

References

Smedema JP, Snoep G, van Kroonenburgh MP, et al: Evaluation of the accuracy of gadolinium-enhanced cardiovascular magnetic resonance in the diagnosis of cardiac sarcoidosis, *J Am Coll Cardiol* 45(10):1683–1690, 2005.

Youssef G, Beanlands RS, Birnie DH, Nery PB: Cardiac sarcoidosis: applications of imaging in diagnosis and directing treatment, *Heart* 97(24):2078–2087, 2011.

Cross-Reference

Cardiac Imaging: The REQUISITES, ed 3, pp 89, 92.

Comment

Imaging

Short-axis and four-chamber images show patchy late gadolinium enhancement that does not follow a typical vascular distribution and spares the subendocardial layer (Figs. A-C). T2-weighted black blood short-axis image shows no hyperintensity to indicate active inflammation (Fig. D). This patient had pulmonary sarcoidosis and was given a presumptive diagnosis of cardiac sarcoidosis based on the MRI findings.

Epidemiology

Myocardial involvement by sarcoidosis is uncommon, clinically affecting approximately 5% of all patients with the disease. Autopsy series show cardiac involvement in 27% of asymptomatic patients. The cardiovascular system is the third most commonly affected organ system. When the heart is involved, patients may be asymptomatic but are at greater risk for acute heart failure, arrhythmia, and sudden cardiac death. Sarcoidosis most commonly affects the myocardium; specifically, there is often sparing of the subendocardium with involvement of the basal septum, left ventricular free wall, and right ventricular free wall.

Notes

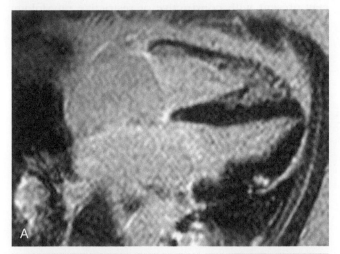

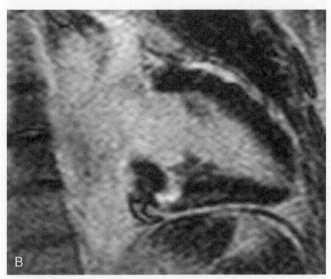

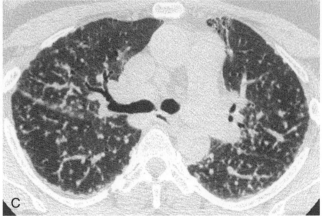

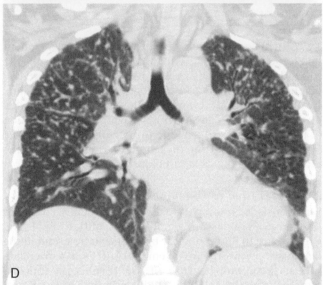

History: A 45-year-old man presents with a new arrhythmia and chronic lung disease.

1. What should be included in the differential diagnosis for the cardiac findings? (Choose all that apply.)
   A. Myocarditis
   B. Infarction
   C. Ischemia
   D. Athlete's heart
   E. Sarcoidosis

2. What is the high-resolution chest CT finding?
   A. Nodules
   B. Masses
   C. Mosaic attenuation
   D. Tracheobronchomalacia

3. Which pattern best describes the distribution of the lung nodules?
   A. Random
   B. Tree-in-bud
   C. Perilymphatic
   D. Centrilobular

4. What is the likely diagnosis?
   A. Myocarditis
   B. Hypertrophic cardiomyopathy
   C. Sarcoidosis
   D. Amyloidosis

CASE 76

Cardiac and Pulmonary Sarcoidosis

1. A and E

2. A

3. C

4. C

References

Smedema JP, Snoep G, van Kroonenburgh MP, et al: Evaluation of the accuracy of gadolinium-enhanced cardiovascular magnetic resonance in the diagnosis of cardiac sarcoidosis, *J Am Coll Cardiol* 45(10):1683–1690, 2005.

Youssef G, Beanlands RS, Birnie DH, et al: Cardiac sarcoidosis: applications of imaging in diagnosis and directing treatment, *Heart* 97(24):2078–2087, 2011.

Cross-Reference

Cardiac Imaging: The REQUISITES, ed 3, pp 89, 92.

Comment

Imaging

Two inversion recovery late gadolinium enhancement images show nodular enhancing foci that spare the subendocardium (Figs. A and B). The main differential diagnostic considerations include several nonischemic cardiomyopathies (i.e., myocarditis, sarcoidosis, amyloidosis). Chest CT scan shows a perilymphatic distribution of lung nodules with a mid to upper zone predominance (Figs. C and D). Putting these two findings together, the most likely diagnosis is sarcoidosis.

Modalities Used to Diagnose Myocardial Sarcoidosis

Sarcoidosis is an idiopathic disease characterized by the presence of noncaseating granulomas. MRI, PET/CT, and gallium and thallium nuclear imaging can be useful in the diagnosis of cardiac involvement. MRI is a particularly robust technique because of the absence of ionizing radiation and the ability to guide endomyocardial biopsy to appropriate areas of active disease. MRI can assess treatment response after initiation of corticosteroids or immunomodulator therapy.

Diagnosis

The diagnosis is difficult in the absence of known pulmonary sarcoidosis. MRI findings of active disease include patchy and nodular T2 hyperintensity with focal wall thickening and late gadolinium enhancement in involved myocardium. Scarring, fibrosis, and wall thinning identify the chronic form of disease. The patchy myocardial enhancement in sarcoidosis often spares the subendocardium and does not follow a vascular distribution.

Cardiomyopathy

Myocardial sarcoidosis can cause a restrictive cardiomyopathy. The left ventricular myocardium has increased stiffness (reduced compliance) leading to poor diastolic filling and reduced cardiac output. Systolic function is often preserved or mildly decreased. Clinically, patients may present with constrictive or restrictive physiology with dyspnea on exertion, lower extremity edema, ascites, and equalization of cardiac chamber pressures. MRI can differentiate restrictive cardiomyopathy from constrictive pericarditis. Constrictive pericarditis often has pericardial thickening measuring greater than 4 mm. Potential causes of restrictive cardiomyopathy include sarcoidosis and amyloidosis; restrictive cardiomyopathy can also be idiopathic.

Notes

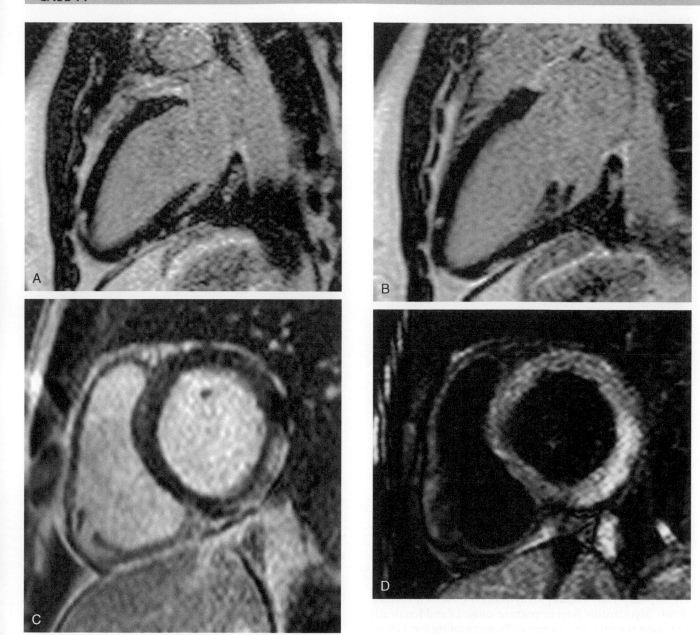

History: A 19-year-old man with a 1-week history of fevers and upper respiratory tract symptoms presents with chest pain and an elevated troponin value.

1. What could cause this pattern of late gadolinium enhancement? (Choose all that apply.)
   A. Pericarditis
   B. Myocarditis
   C. Amyloidosis
   D. Sarcoidosis
   E. Infarction

2. What sequence is shown in Fig. D?
   A. Phase contrast
   B. Steady-state free precession (SSFP)
   C. Double inversion recovery
   D. Single inversion recovery

3. What is the likely diagnosis given the patient history and imaging findings?
   A. Pericarditis
   B. Myocarditis
   C. Sarcoidosis
   D. Myocardial infarction

4. What is the gold standard for diagnosing this entity?
   A. Echocardiography
   B. MRI
   C. Troponin
   D. Biopsy

CASE 77

Myocarditis

1. B, C, and D

2. C

3. B

4. D

References

Deux JF, Maatouk M, Lim P, et al: Acute myocarditis: diagnostic value of contrast-enhanced cine steady-state free precession MRI sequences, *AJR Am J Roentgenol* 197(5):1081–1087, 2011.

Feldman AM, McNamara D: Myocarditis, *N Engl J Med* 343(19):1388–1398, 2000.

Cross-Reference

Cardiac Imaging: The REQUISITES, ed 3, pp 91–92, 292–294.

Comment

Imaging

Inversion recovery late gadolinium enhancement images show nodular enhancement sparing the endocardium in the left ventricle, which does not correspond to a vascular distribution (Figs. A-C). T2-weighted black blood imaging shows hyperintensity along the inferior and lateral ventricular walls corresponding to the site of late gadolinium enhancement (Fig. D).

Epidemiology and Symptoms

Myocarditis is an inflammatory disease of the myocardium, which in the United States most commonly follows a viral infection. It occurs as secondary to the virus itself or as an immune-mediated response to viral antigens. Other causes of myocarditis include bacterial and parasitic infections and certain cardiotoxic drugs (i.e., anthracyclines and trastuzumab). Chagas disease is the most common cause worldwide. Most patients are relatively asymptomatic, and the diagnosis is discovered in postmortem studies. Symptomatic patients present with chest pain, heart failure, arrhythmia, or sudden cardiac death. Myocarditis is an important cause of sudden death in young patients (<40 years old), accounting for 12% to 20% of cases.

Diagnosis with MRI

MRI is a useful imaging modality in patients with suspected myocarditis. The acute and subacute phases of disease are characterized by T2 hyperintensity within involved myocardium (Fig. D). There is usually no late gadolinium enhancement unless irreversible damage has occurred (Figs. A-C). Early abnormalities predominate in the epicardial left ventricular free wall, the interventricular septum, and occasionally the right ventricle. Late gadolinium enhancement signifies irreversible damage or fibrosis. Specific patterns of enhancement include patchy, diffuse, nodular, or transmural, which does not follow a typical vascular territory.

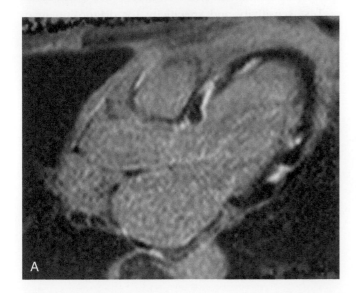

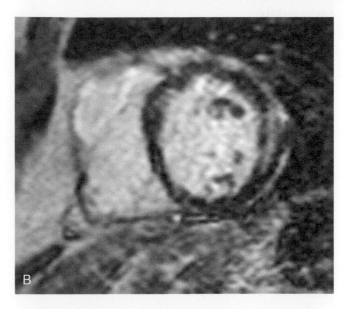

History: A 60-year-old woman presents with dyspnea on exertion and chest pain.

1. What should be included in the differential diagnosis? (Choose all that apply.)
   A. Amyloidosis
   B. Myocarditis
   C. Infarction
   D. Sarcoidosis

2. What is the most likely diagnosis in the presence of paratracheal and symmetric hilar lymphadenopathy?
   A. Amyloidosis
   B. Myocarditis
   C. Myocardial infarction
   D. Sarcoidosis

3. What is the most likely diagnosis if the patient's chest radiograph was clear and her chest pain started after a viral illness?
   A. Amyloidosis
   B. Myocarditis
   C. Infarction
   D. Sarcoidosis

4. What is the significance of late gadolinium enhancement in myocarditis?
   A. Fibrosis
   B. Capillary leak
   C. Hyperemia
   D. Edema

CASE 78

Myocarditis

1. A, B, and D

2. D

3. B

4. A

References

Deux JF, Maatouk M, Lim P, et al: Acute myocarditis: diagnostic value of contrast-enhanced cine steady-state free precession MRI sequences, *AJR Am J Roentgenol* 197(5):1081-1087, 2011.

Feldman AM, McNamara D: Myocarditis, *N Engl J Med* 343(19):1388-1398, 2000.

Friedrich MG, Sechtem U, Schulz-Menger J, et al: Cardiovascular magnetic resonance in myocarditis: a JACC White Paper, *J Am Coll Cardiol* 53(17):1475-1487, 2009.

Cross-Reference

Cardiac Imaging: The REQUISITES, ed 3, pp 91-92, 292-294.

Comment

Imaging

Late gadolinium enhancement four-chamber and short-axis images show patchy enhancement in the left ventricle with sparing of the endocardium (Figs. A and B). The differential diagnosis includes myocarditis or sarcoidosis. Amyloidosis is possible if the patient presented with symptoms of restrictive cardiomyopathy. This patient was diagnosed with myocarditis after excluding sarcoidosis.

Description

Myocarditis represents inflammation of myocardial tissue. It most commonly follows a viral infection and is usually seen in previously healthy patients. It is an important cause of sudden cardiac death in young patients and is a recognized cause of dilated cardiomyopathy. Endomyocardial biopsy is considered the gold standard for diagnosis, but it is invasive and may be negative owing to sampling error.

Diagnosis with MRI

MRI is a noninvasive technique that aids in the diagnosis of myocarditis in the correct clinical setting. MRI identifies the disease in 30% of patients with chest pain, elevated troponin, and clinically normal coronary arteries. There are three findings that occur with myocarditis:

1. T2 hyperintensity indicates inflammation and edema. This is potentially reversible in the setting of no late gadolinium enhancement.
2. Early gadolinium enhancement obtained minutes after gadolinium injection indicates hyperemia and capillary leak.
3. Late gadolinium enhancement is patchy and does not correspond to a typical vascular distribution. It indicates irreversible injury with necrosis and fibrosis.

Test sensitivity and specificity for diagnosing myocarditis increase with more positive findings (i.e., T2 hyperintensity, early gadolinium enhancement, and late gadolinium enhancement).

Prognosis

Late gadolinium enhancement occurring 4 weeks after the acute episode has shown prognostic value in predicting poor functional and clinical outcomes. A reduced ejection fraction and right ventricular involvement are echocardiographic markers of an increased risk for sudden cardiac death and future need for cardiac transplantation. Patients with myocarditis are usually treated supportively with heart failure and arrhythmia management. Immunosuppressive therapy is initiated when myocarditis results from an autoimmune disease.

Notes

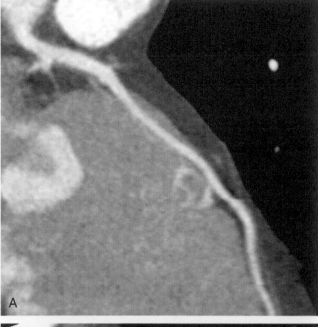

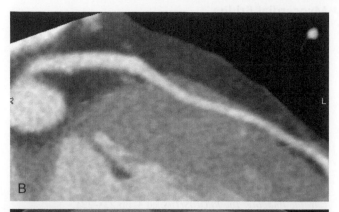

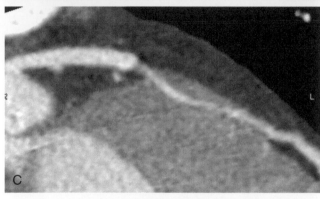

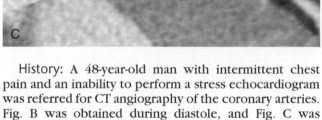

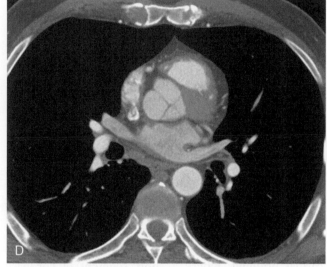

History: A 48-year-old man with intermittent chest pain and an inability to perform a stress echocardiogram was referred for CT angiography of the coronary arteries. Fig. B was obtained during diastole, and Fig. C was obtained during early systole.

1. What are considered risk factors for developing coronary artery disease? (Choose all that apply.)
   A. Moderate exercise
   B. Hypertension
   C. Mantle radiation
   D. Dyslipidemia

2. What is the finding in Fig. B obtained in diastole and in Fig. C obtained in systole?
   A. Fixed stenosis
   B. Dynamic stenosis
   C. Calcified plaque
   D. Noncalcified plaque

3. What is the diagnosis?
   A. Atherosclerosis
   B. Coronary artery spasm
   C. Myocardial bridge
   D. Dissection

4. What is the most common treatment for this lesion?
   A. Beta blocker
   B. Percutaneous stent
   C. Surgical resection of bridged segment
   D. No treatment

Myocardial Bridge

1. B, C, and D

2. B

3. C

4. D

Reference

Möhlenkamp S, Hort W, Ge J, et al: Update on myocardial bridging, *Circulation* 106(20):2616-2622, 2002.

Cross-Reference

Cardiac Imaging: The REQUISITES, ed 3, pp 223-224.

Comment

Imaging

Multiple images from CT angiography of the coronary arteries show a myocardial bridge affecting the mid left anterior descending coronary artery (Figs. A-D). An image obtained during diastole shows no narrowing (Fig. B). An image obtained during systole shows circumferential narrowing (Fig. C). On further questioning, this patient had intermittent chest pain not induced by exercise, and the myocardial bridge was deemed an incidental finding.

Description

The coronary arteries normally course along the surface of the heart through epicardial fat. Approximately 25% of patients have an intramyocardial course, termed myocardial bridging, where a short segment of coronary artery is completely surrounded by myocardium. During systole, there is compression of the bridged coronary artery (Fig. C). Because most blood flow (approximately two thirds) occurs during diastole (Fig. B), this compression rarely results in symptoms. Myocardial bridging most commonly affects the midsegment of the left anterior descending coronary artery as in this case.

Treatment

Myocardial bridging is usually an incidental finding of minimal or no clinical significance. Uncommonly, bridging may cause angina, left ventricular dysfunction, or myocardial infarction. Clinical symptoms are more likely if the bridged segment is long or the dynamic stenosis also occurs in early diastole. The available treatment options for symptomatic patients are beta blockers, percutaneous stenting, and surgical resection of the muscle bridge.

Notes

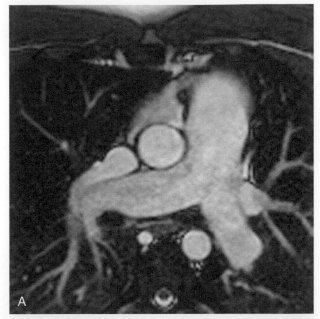

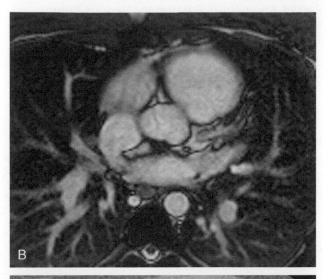

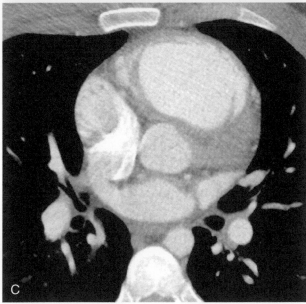

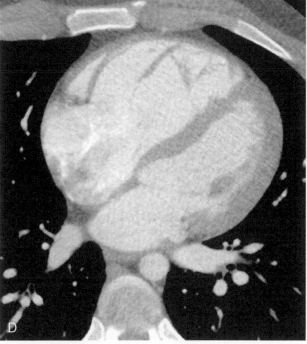

History: A 19-year-old man presents with lightheadedness and syncope after football practice.

1. What should be included in the differential diagnosis for a left-to-right shunt? (Choose all that apply.)
   A. Partial anomalous pulmonary venous return (PAPVR)
   B. Atrial septal defect (ASD)
   C. Eisenmenger syndrome
   D. Tetralogy of Fallot

2. What is the cardiac finding?
   A. ASD
   B. Ventricular septal defect
   C. Patent foramen ovale
   D. Anomalous coronary artery

3. What is the most likely cause of the right atrial and ventricular enlargement in this patient?
   A. Left heart failure
   B. Primary pulmonary hypertension
   C. Left-to-right shunt
   D. Chronic lung disease

4. What is the pulmonary finding?
   A. Anomalous pulmonary venous return
   B. Pulmonary mass
   C. Pulmonary embolism
   D. Hilar lymphadenopathy

Partial Anomalous Pulmonary Venous Return and Atrial Septal Defect

1. A and B

2. A

3. C

4. A

References

Hijii T, Fukushige J, Hara T: Diagnosis and management of partial anomalous pulmonary venous connection: a review of 28 pediatric cases, *Cardiology* 89(2):148-151, 1998.

Ho ML, Bhalla S, Bierhals A, et al: MDCT of partial anomalous pulmonary venous return (PAPVR) in adults, *J Thorac Imaging* 24(2):89-95, 2009.

Cross-Reference

Cardiac Imaging: The REQUISITES, ed 3, pp 330-335.

Comment

Imaging

MRI shows anomalous drainage of a portion of the right lung into the superior vena cava (Fig. A). PAPVR is an atrial level shunt. Images of the heart (Figs. B and C) show a defect in the interatrial septum located posteriorly and superiorly, which is consistent with a sinus venosus ASD. This patient had a large left-to-right shunt (Fig. D) and underwent surgical correction with ASD patching and redirection of the anomalous pulmonary veins into the left circulation.

Associations

PAPVR may be associated with other congenital abnormalities, most commonly a sinus venosus ASD (sinus venosus defect). Patients can be asymptomatic but may present with dyspnea, exercise intolerance, pulmonary hypertension, or syncope depending on the degree of shunt. The indications for surgical correction are symptoms or a large shunt (i.e., pulmonary blood flow twice that of systemic blood flow). Magnetic resonance angiography (MRA) can accurately depict the presence, size, and location of the PAPVR and ASD. MRI can quantify the shunt fraction and help determine the ideal timing to perform surgery.

Notes

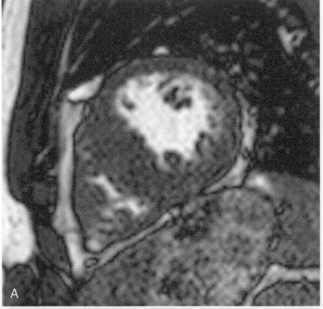

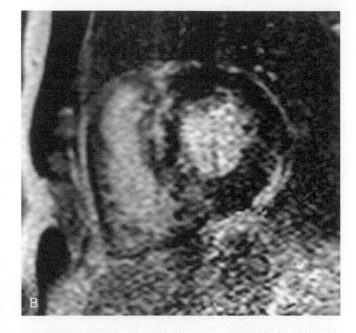

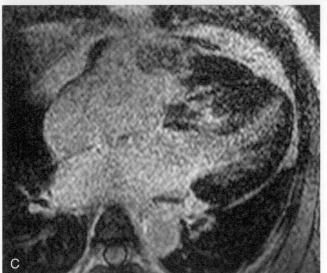

History: A patient presents with heart failure.

1. What should be included in the differential diagnosis for the pattern of late gadolinium enhancement shown in Figs. B and C? (Choose all that apply.)
   A. Myocarditis
   B. Cardiomyopathy
   C. Hibernating myocardium
   D. Myocardial infarction

2. Based on the images, what is the most likely diagnosis?
   A. Sarcoidosis
   B. Amyloidosis
   C. Dilated cardiomyopathy
   D. Hypertrophic cardiomyopathy (HCM)

3. What is the distribution of hypertrophy in this patient?
   A. Concentric
   B. Septal
   C. Midventricular
   D. Apical

4. Which of the following is the least appropriate treatment for this patient?
   A. Medical management
   B. Ethanol septal ablation
   C. Surgery
   D. Heart transplant

Hypertrophic Cardiomyopathy

1. A and B

2. D

3. B

4. D

References

Harris SR, Glockner J, Misselt AJ, et al: Cardiac MR imaging of nonischemic cardiomyopathies, *Magn Reson Imaging Clin N Am* 16(2):165–183, 2008.

Soler R, Rodriguez E, Remuinan C, et al: Magnetic resonance imaging of primary cardiomyopathies, *J Comput Assist Tomogr* 27(5):724–734, 2003.

Cross-Reference

Cardiac Imaging: The REQUISITES, ed 3, pp 53, 284–288.

Comment

Etiology and Clinical Features

HCM is inherited as an autosomal dominant trait with variable penetrance. Patients may be asymptomatic, or they may present with atrial fibrillation, heart failure, syncope, or sudden cardiac death, which is the leading cause of mortality in these patients. Asymmetric hypertrophy of the ventricular septum is the most common distribution, seen in 90% of patients with HCM. Other patterns of hypertrophy are right ventricular, left ventricular, septal, apical, midventricular, and concentric. Patients with heart failure secondary to significant septal hypertrophy and left ventricular outflow obstruction can be treated with septal myectomy or percutaneous transluminal septal myocardial ablation with ethanol.

MRI

MRI can provide anatomic and functional information in HCM and can be most useful when the diagnosis is in question, when invasive therapy is being considered, or when clinical concern requires more thorough assessment than that provided by echocardiography. MRI can be used to identify the distribution of thickened myocardium, to evaluate for systolic anterior motion of the mitral valve, and to calculate left ventricular mass (Fig. A). Late gadolinium enhancement MRI characteristically shows patchy midmyocardial enhancement (Figs. B and C). MRI also can be used for functional evaluation of left ventricular outflow tract obstruction.

Notes

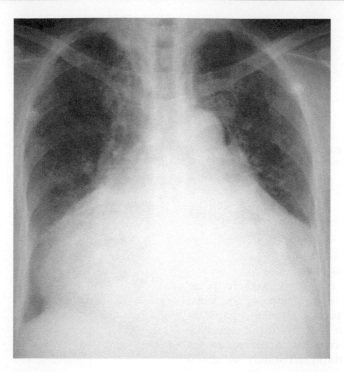

History: A patient presents with dyspnea.

1. What should be included in the differential diagnosis? (Choose all that apply.)
   A. Tricuspid regurgitation
   B. Mitral regurgitation
   C. Dilated cardiomyopathy
   D. Pericardial effusion

2. What is this appearance called?
   A. Water-bottle heart
   B. Boot-shaped heart
   C. Box-shaped heart
   D. Wall-to-wall heart

3. What is the most likely diagnosis?
   A. Tricuspid regurgitation
   B. Mitral regurgitation
   C. Dilated cardiomyopathy
   D. Pericardial effusion

4. Which imaging modality best assesses the valve leaflets?
   A. Echocardiography
   B. CT scan
   C. MRI
   D. Angiography

CASE 82

Tricuspid Regurgitation

1. A, C, and D

2. D

3. A

4. A

Reference

Walker CM, Reddy GP, Steiner RM: Radiology of the heart. In Rosendorff C, editor: *Essential Cardiology*, ed 3, New York, 2013, Springer.

Cross-Reference

Cardiac Imaging: The REQUISITES, ed 3, pp 205–206.

Comment

Pathology, Etiology, and Treatment

Tricuspid regurgitation can occur when there is an abnormality of one or more components of the valve apparatus: the anulus, leaflets, chordae, papillary muscles, and right ventricular wall. Tricuspid regurgitation can be acquired or congenital. Acquired causes include pulmonary hypertension secondary to mitral valve disease (most common cause), papillary muscle rupture, rheumatic heart disease, bacterial endocarditis, and carcinoid syndrome. The most common congenital cause is Ebstein anomaly. When tricuspid regurgitation is secondary to mitral valve disease, treatment of the mitral disease can relieve the tricuspid regurgitation. In more severe cases, tricuspid valve replacement or annuloplasty is performed.

Imaging

Chest radiographs demonstrate marked enlargement of the right atrium and ventricle (Figure). The heart can become massively enlarged, resulting in the so-called wall-to-wall heart. The differential diagnosis includes tricuspid regurgitation, dilated cardiomyopathy, and pericardial effusion. Echocardiography is performed to evaluate regurgitation further. Angiography and MRI can also be performed in selected cases. MRI is highly accurate for quantification of the severity of regurgitation.

Notes

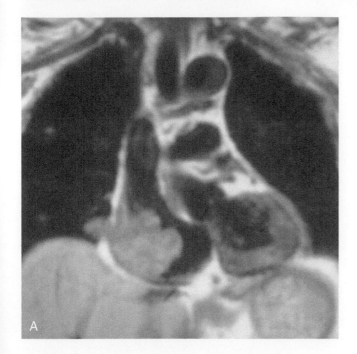

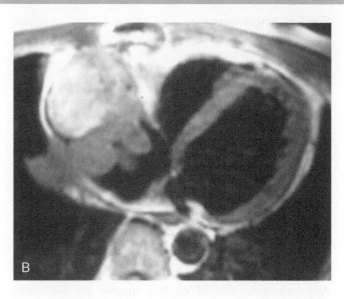

History: A patient presents with chest pain.

1. What should be included in the differential diagnosis? (Choose all that apply.)
   A. Metastasis
   B. Lipoma
   C. Myxoma
   D. Angiosarcoma

2. What is the most common mass in the heart?
   A. Thrombus
   B. Myxoma
   C. Metastasis
   D. Angiosarcoma

3. Which chamber is involved?
   A. Left atrium
   B. Left ventricle
   C. Right atrium
   D. Right ventricle

4. If this is a primary tumor, what is the most likely diagnosis?
   A. Myxoma
   B. Angiosarcoma
   C. Rhabdomyosarcoma
   D. Rhabdomyoma

Cardiac Angiosarcoma

1. A and D

2. A

3. C

4. B

Reference

Randhawa K, Ganeshan A, Hoey ET: Magnetic resonance imaging of cardiac tumors: part 2, malignant tumors and tumor-like conditions, *Curr Probl Diagn Radiol* 40(4):169–179, 2011.

Cross-Reference

Cardiac Imaging: The REQUISITES, ed 3, pp 281–282.

Comment

Pathology, Etiology, and Treatment

Approximately 98% of cardiac tumors are secondary tumors. The most common malignant primary cardiac tumor is angiosarcoma. Other primary malignant tumors are rare and include rhabdomyosarcoma, leiomyosarcoma, liposarcoma, and lymphoma. Definitive diagnosis is made with endomyocardial or open biopsy.

MRI

MRI can show tumor size and location and cardiac function. Contrast-enhanced sequences can delineate tumor margins and invasion into adjacent structures. The presence of enhancement does not signify malignancy; benign tumors enhance too. Features that suggest a primary malignant cardiac tumor include irregular or ill-defined margination, invasiveness, extension outside the heart (Figs. A and B), involvement of more than one chamber, central necrosis, large pericardial effusion, and lung nodules—which raise the possibility of metastases.

Notes

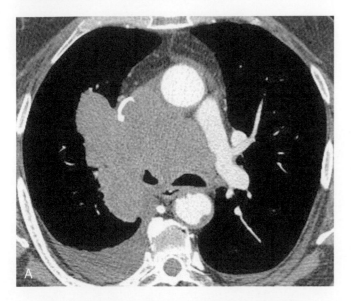

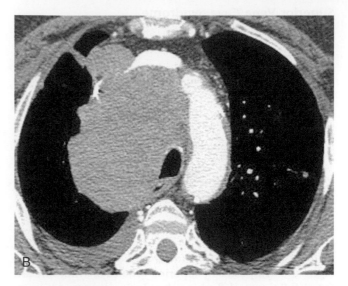

History: A patient presents with facial swelling.

1. What are potential causes of this appearance? (Choose all that apply.)
   A. Fibrosing mediastinitis
   B. Lymphoma
   C. Angiosarcoma
   D. Lung cancer

2. Which vessel is most severely narrowed?
   A. Azygos vein
   B. Superior vena cava
   C. Descending aorta
   D. Ascending aorta

3. What is the most likely diagnosis?
   A. Fibrosing mediastinitis
   B. Lymphoma
   C. Angiosarcoma
   D. Lung cancer

4. What is the most appropriate treatment in the acute setting?
   A. Chemotherapy
   B. Radiation therapy
   C. Stent
   D. Surgery

Superior Vena Cava Syndrome

1. B, C, and D

2. B

3. D

4. B

References

Sheth S, Ebert MD, Fishman EK: Superior vena cava obstruction evaluation with MDCT, *AJR Am J Roentgenol* 194(4):W336–W346, 2010.

Wilson LD, Detterbeck FC, Yahalom J: Clinical practice. Superior vena cava syndrome with malignant causes, *N Engl J Med* 356(18):1862–1869, 2007.

Comment

Clinical Presentation and Etiology

Signs and symptoms of superior vena cava syndrome are facial fullness and flushing, headache, upper extremity edema, and prominence of veins in the face and upper chest. The acute manifestation can be life-threatening. Most cases occur secondary to bronchogenic cancer. Other causes include fibrosing mediastinitis (most commonly secondary to histoplasmosis), lymphoma, other malignant tumors, and superior vena cava thrombosis.

Imaging

CT can be performed to assess the mediastinum and to demonstrate the narrowing of the superior vena cava (Figs. A and B). MRI also can be performed to evaluate venous stenosis or occlusion and to identify the cause of narrowing.

Notes

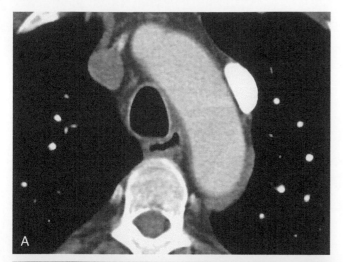

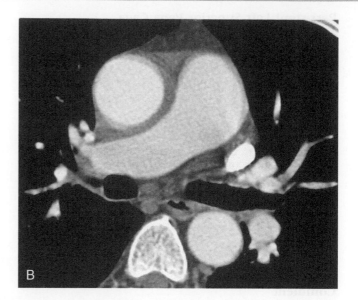

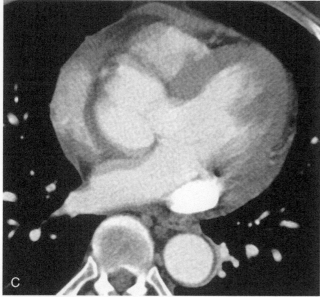

History: No patient history is available.

1. What should be included in the differential diagnosis of the vessel to the left of the aortic arch in Fig. A? (Choose all that apply.)
   A. Superior intercostal vein
   B. Hemiazygos vein
   C. Persistent left superior vena cava (SVC)
   D. Vertical vein

2. Taking into account all the figures, what is the most likely diagnosis?
   A. Superior intercostal vein
   B. Hemiazygos vein
   C. Persistent left SVC
   D. Vertical vein

3. What structure most commonly connects the right SVC and left SVC?
   A. Bridging vein
   B. Right brachiocephalic vein
   C. Coronary sinus
   D. Right atrium

4. Which other anomaly occurs in most patients with persistent left SVC?
   A. No other anomaly
   B. Atrioventricular septal defect
   C. Tetralogy of Fallot
   D. Single ventricle

CASE 85

Persistent Left Superior Vena Cava

1. C and D

2. C

3. A

4. A

References

Burney K, Young H, Barnard SA, et al: CT appearances of congenital and acquired abnormalities of the superior vena cava, *Clin Radiol* 62(9):837-842, 2007.

Uçar O, Paşaoğlu L, Ciçekçioğlu H, et al: Persistent left superior vena cava with absent right superior vena cava: a case report and review of the literature, *Cardiovasc J Afr* 21(3):164-166, 2010.

Cross-Reference

Cardiac Imaging: The REQUISITES, ed 3, pp 27-29.

Comment

Etiology

Persistent left SVC results when the left anterior cardinal vein persists after birth. The left brachiocephalic vein drains into the left SVC, which usually connects to the coronary sinus. The coronary sinus may be dilated from the increase in flow, especially if there is no right SVC. Most individuals are asymptomatic, and their anatomy is otherwise normal. Most individuals with a persistent left SVC have a right SVC as well—hence the designation "duplicated SVC."

Associated Anomalies

Rarely, the left SVC drains into the left atrium. In this situation, multiple severe cardiac anomalies may coexist, such as common atrium, atrioventricular canal defect, single ventricle, asplenia, and polysplenia. Persistent left SVC is also associated with atrial septal defect, tetralogy of Fallot, and partial and total anomalous pulmonary venous connection.

Imaging

Persistent left SVC may come to light after placement of a central venous catheter, pulmonary artery catheter, or pacemaker. The anomaly may be seen incidentally on CT (Figs. A-C) or MRI, which can demonstrate a round or oval vessel to the left of the aortic arch.

Notes

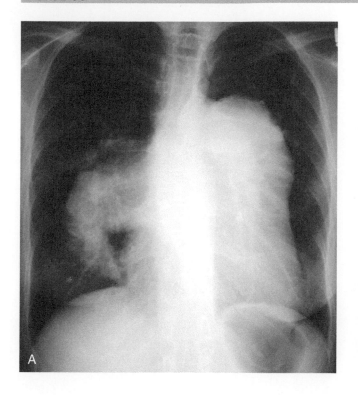

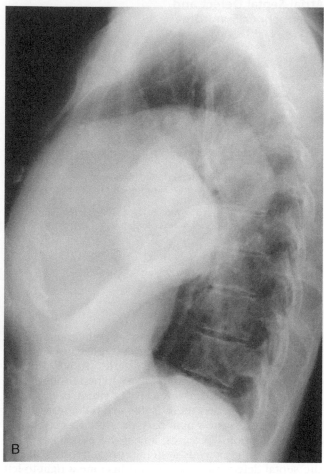

History: A patient presents with fatigue.

1. What should be included in the differential diagnosis? (Choose all that apply.)
   A. Sleep apnea
   B. Pulmonary fibrosis
   C. Chronic thromboembolism
   D. Atrial septal defect

2. This patient is acyanotic and has a shunt lesion. What is the most likely diagnosis?
   A. Atrial septal defect
   B. Ventricular septal defect
   C. Atrioventricular septal defect
   D. Patent ductus arteriosus

3. Which of the following is not characteristic of Eisenmenger syndrome?
   A. Cyanosis
   B. Paradoxical embolism
   C. Decreased pulmonary vascularity
   D. Left-to-right shunt

4. Which pulmonary-to-systemic flow ratio (Qp:Qs) is characteristic of Eisenmenger syndrome?
   A. 0.7:1
   B. 1:1
   C. 1.5:1
   D. 3:1

Atrial Septal Defect and Eisenmenger Syndrome

1. A, C, and D

2. A

3. D

4. A

References

Diller GP, Gatzoulis MA: Pulmonary vascular disease in adults with congenital heart disease, *Circulation* 115(8):1039-1050, 2007.

Walker CM, Reddy GP, Steiner RM: Radiology of the heart. In Rosendorff C, editor: *Essential Cardiology*, ed 3, New York, 2013, Springer.

Wang ZJ, Reddy GP, Gotway MB, et al: Cardiovascular shunts: MR imaging evaluation, *Radiographics* 23(Spec No):S181–S194, 2003.

Cross-Reference

Cardiac Imaging: The REQUISITES, ed 3, pp 16–18.

Comment

Etiology and Clinical Implications

When an atrial septal defect is long-standing, pulmonary pressure can increase dramatically and cause marked enlargement of the pulmonary arteries. Although there are numerous causes of pulmonary hypertension, it has been reported that an intracardiac shunt is the most common cause when there is massive pulmonary artery enlargement. As the pulmonary pressure increases, left-to-right shunting decreases, and if the pulmonary pressure eventually exceeds systemic pressure, flow across the septal defect can reverse and become a right-to-left shunt; this is known as Eisenmenger syndrome. In the setting of Eisenmenger syndrome, patients may be cyanotic, and paradoxical embolism can result in a transient ischemic attack or a stroke.

Imaging

Radiographs can demonstrate marked enlargement of the central pulmonary arteries, consistent with pulmonary arterial hypertension (Figs. A and B). The pulmonary vascularity is typically decreased in the setting of Eisenmenger syndrome. Velocity-encoded cine MRI can be performed to obtain the Qp:Qs and quantify the severity of the shunt.

Notes

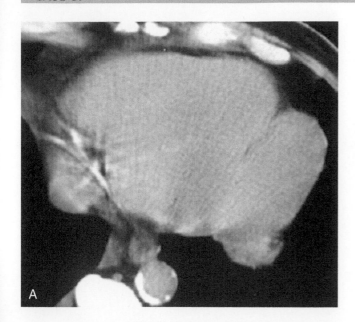

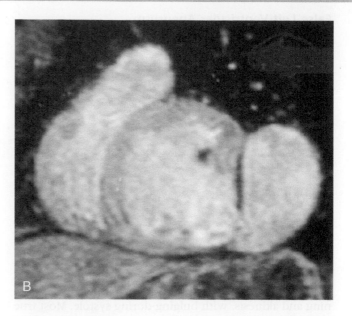

History: A patient is referred for CT-guided fine-needle aspiration of a mass seen on chest radiographs.

1. What should be included in the differential diagnosis based on Fig. A? (Choose all that apply.)
   A. Lung cancer
   B. Metastasis
   C. Ventricular aneurysm
   D. Pericardial cyst

2. What is the most likely diagnosis based on Fig. B?
   A. Lung cancer
   B. Metastasis
   C. Ventricular aneurysm
   D. Pericardial cyst

3. Which of the following features is most specific for the MRI diagnosis of a false aneurysm?
   A. Inferodiaphragmatic location
   B. Disruption of the ventricular wall
   C. Narrow ostium
   D. Large size

4. What is the most appropriate management of a false aneurysm?
   A. No therapy
   B. Medical management
   C. Stent graft
   D. Surgery

False Left Ventricular Aneurysm

1. B, C, and D

2. C

3. C

4. D

Reference

White RD: MR and CT assessment for ischemic cardiac disease, *J Magn Reson Imaging* 19(6):659-675, 2004.

Cross-Reference

Cardiac Imaging: The REQUISITES, ed 3, pp 236-237.

Comment

Pathology and Etiology

Left ventricular aneurysms result from transmural myocardial infarction. True aneurysms have focal wall thinning and akinesis, with bulging during systole. Most true aneurysms are located in the anteroapical region of the left ventricle and have wide necks. A false aneurysm represents a contained rupture. Most false aneurysms are inferoposterior in location and are connected to the left ventricle via a narrow neck.

Treatment

True aneurysms are usually managed medically unless there is substantial dysfunction, such as heart failure, arrhythmia, or peripheral embolization of thrombus. False aneurysms are usually resected because of the high risk of rupture.

Imaging and Diagnostic Criteria

True and false aneurysms can be differentiated on the basis of their necks on MRI or CT (Figs. A and B). Location is suggestive but not definitive for differentiating a true aneurysm from a false aneurysm. The inferoposterior location of the aneurysm and the narrow neck (<50% of the diameter of the aneurysm) indicate a false aneurysm.

Notes

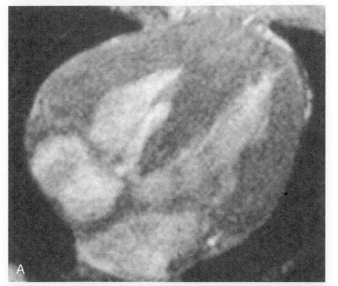

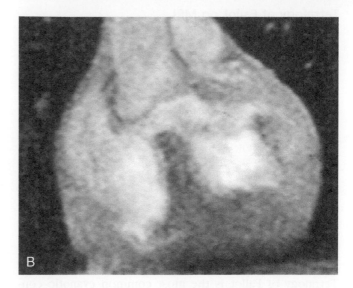

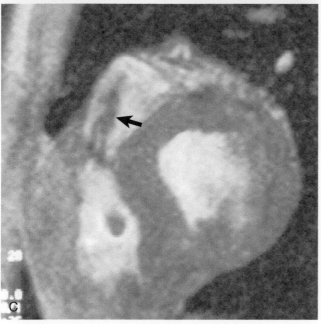

History: A patient presents with cyanosis.

1. What findings are seen? (Choose all that apply.)
   A. Right ventricular hypertrophy
   B. Overriding aorta
   C. Pulmonary infundibular stenosis
   D. Ventricular septal defect

2. What is the most likely diagnosis?
   A. Atrioventricular septal defect
   B. Tetralogy of Fallot
   C. Transposition of the great arteries
   D. Pulmonary atresia with ventricular septal defect

3. What is a common complication of surgery for tetralogy of Fallot?
   A. Overriding aorta
   B. Right ventricular rupture
   C. Pulmonary stenosis
   D. Pulmonary regurgitation

4. What artifact is indicated by the arrow in Fig. C?
   A. Spin dephasing
   B. Aliasing
   C. Susceptibility
   D. Phase wrap

Tetralogy of Fallot on MRI

1. A, B, C, and D

2. B

3. D

4. A

Reference

Reddy GP, Higgins CB: Magnetic resonance imaging of congenital heart disease: evaluation of morphology and function, *Semin Roentgenol* 38(4):342-351, 2003.

Cross-Reference

Cardiac Imaging: The REQUISITES, ed 3, pp 359–367.

Comment

Anomalies of Tetralogy of Fallot

Tetralogy of Fallot is the most common cyanotic congenital heart disease. The four primary lesions of tetralogy of Fallot are an overriding aorta, ventricular septal defect, pulmonary infundibular stenosis, and right ventricular hypertrophy. Pulmonary stenosis can be present at multiple levels, including infundibular (most common), valvular, supravalvular, and peripheral. Approximately 25% of patients with tetralogy of Fallot have a right aortic arch, usually a mirror-image arch.

MRI

MRI can be performed for comprehensive evaluation of tetralogy of Fallot (Figs. A-C). Contrast-enhanced magnetic resonance angiography (MRA) can show the pulmonary artery sizes and can identify peripheral pulmonary arterial stenoses. Velocity-encoded cine phase contrast images can be obtained to measure differential right and left pulmonary flow and to quantify regurgitation in the postoperative setting. Cine MRI is employed for the quantitative appraisal of right ventricular function after surgery.

Notes

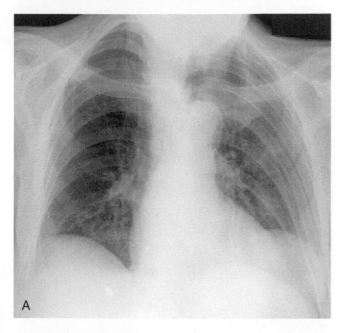

A

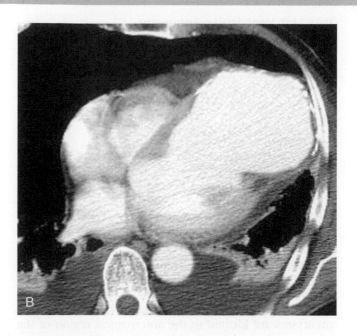

B

History: A patient presents with dyspnea on exertion.

1. What should be included in the differential diagnosis based on Fig. A? (Choose all that apply.)
   A. Lung cancer
   B. Ventricular aneurysm
   C. Pericardial cyst
   D. Bochdalek hernia

2. What is the most likely diagnosis based on Fig. B?
   A. Lung cancer
   B. Ventricular aneurysm
   C. Pericardial cyst
   D. Bochdalek hernia

3. What characteristic is most specific for the CT diagnosis of a true aneurysm?
   A. Anteroapical location
   B. Calcification along the ventricular wall
   C. Wide ostium
   D. Large size

4. This aneurysm puts the patient at high risk for which of the following complications?
   A. Peripheral embolization
   B. Sudden death
   C. Ventricular rupture
   D. Recurrent myocardial infarction

True Left Ventricular Aneurysm

1. B, C, and D

2. B

3. C

4. A

Reference

White RD: MR and CT assessment for ischemic cardiac disease, *J Magn Reson Imaging* 19(6):659-675, 2004.

Cross-Reference

Cardiac Imaging: The REQUISITES, ed 3, pp 235-237.

Comment

Pathology, Etiology, and Treatment

Left ventricular aneurysms result from transmural myocardial infarction. True aneurysms have focal wall thinning and akinesis, with bulging during systole. Most true aneurysms are located in the anteroapical region of the left ventricle and have wide necks. A false aneurysm represents a contained rupture. Most false aneurysms are inferoposterior in location and are connected to the left ventricle via a narrow ostium. True aneurysms are managed medically, but they can be resected if they cause dysfunction, such as heart failure, arrhythmia, or peripheral embolization. False aneurysms are typically managed surgically.

Imaging Findings and Diagnostic Criteria

Radiographs may show a contour abnormality along the left ventricle (Fig. A). Calcification or thrombus may be present (Fig. B). With MRI or CT, true and false aneurysms can be differentiated on the basis of their ostia. The size of the ostium (>50% of the aneurysm diameter) is the most specific feature of a true aneurysm. A true aneurysm typically has an ostium that is greater than 50% of the aneurysm diameter (Fig. B), whereas a false aneurysm typically has an ostium that is less than 50% of the aneurysm diameter.

Notes

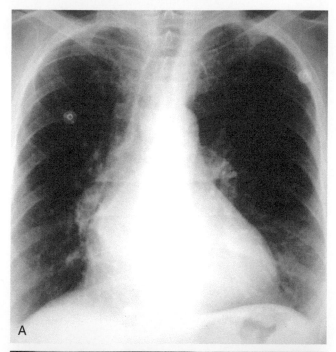

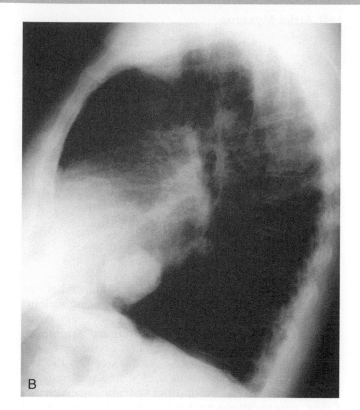

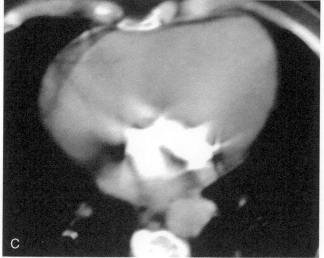

History: A patient presents with heart failure.

1. What should be included in the differential diagnosis? (Choose all that apply.)
   A. Metastasis
   B. Thrombus
   C. Myxoma
   D. Angiosarcoma

2. What is the most common mass in the heart?
   A. Thrombus
   B. Myxoma
   C. Metastasis
   D. Angiosarcoma

3. Which chamber is involved?
   A. Left atrium
   B. Left ventricle
   C. Right atrium
   D. Right ventricle

4. What is the most appropriate management of the mass?
   A. Anticoagulation
   B. Chemotherapy
   C. Radiation therapy
   D. Surgical resection

Left Atrial Myxoma

1. B and C

2. A

3. A

4. D

Reference

Restrepo CS, Largoza A, Lemos DF, et al: CT and MR imaging findings of malignant cardiac tumors, *Curr Probl Diagn Radiol* 34(1):12–21, 2005.

Cross-Reference

Cardiac Imaging: The REQUISITES, ed 3, pp 280–281.

Comment

Clinical Features and Treatment

Myxoma is usually located in the left atrium and is one of the most common benign tumors of the heart. Patients with myxoma can be asymptomatic or develop symptoms of mitral stenosis or constitutional symptoms, including fever, anemia, and elevated erythrocyte sedimentation rate. Embolization of a myxoma to the systemic circulation can occur and can cause transient ischemic attacks, stroke, or other systemic organ disease. Other complications include occlusion of the mitral valve and malignant degeneration. This tumor is usually resected even though it is benign.

Imaging

Myxoma is well circumscribed and often has a narrow pedicle that is attached to the fossa ovalis of the atrial septum. A broad attachment to the atrial wall is less common. Radiographs can show a mass or show nonspecific findings (Figs. A and B). Myxomas can calcify (Fig. C), although dense calcification is uncommon. On black blood MRI, a myxoma typically enhances with administration of a contrast agent. Because of fibrosis, calcification, or iron deposition, myxomas can be dark on steady-state free precession MRI, mimicking the appearance of a thrombus. It is important to look for contrast enhancement on black blood images to differentiate myxoma from a thrombus, which does not enhance.

Notes

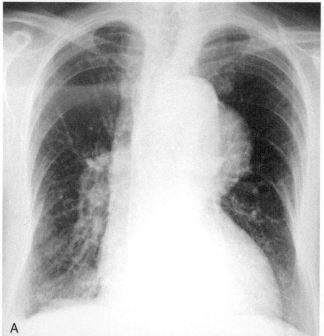

A

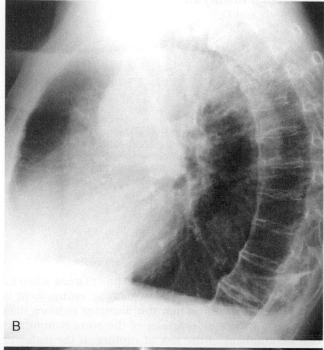

B

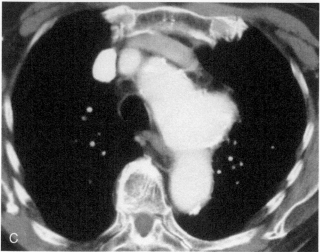

C

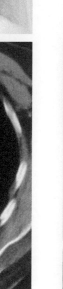

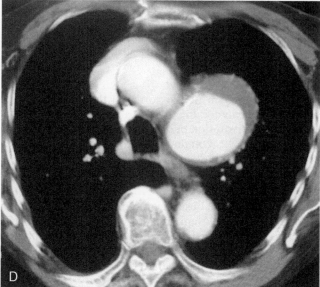

D

History: A patient presents with cough.

1. What should be included in the differential diagnosis based on Figs. A and B? (Choose all that apply.)
   A. Bronchogenic cyst
   B. Lymphadenopathy
   C. Aortic aneurysm
   D. Pulmonary artery aneurysm

2. What is the most likely diagnosis based on Figs. C and D?
   A. Ductus aneurysm
   B. Aortic arch aneurysm
   C. Traumatic pseudoaneurysm
   D. Double aortic arch

3. What is the most common cause of aortic aneurysm?
   A. Annuloaortic ectasia
   B. Syphilis
   C. Takayasu arteritis
   D. Atherosclerosis

4. What is an advantage of MRI over CT for evaluation of the thoracic aorta?
   A. Multiplanar imaging capability
   B. Better spatial resolution
   C. No need for contrast agent
   D. Better imaging in patients with arrhythmia

CASE 91

Aortic Arch Aneurysm

1. A, B, C, and D

2. B

3. D

4. C

Reference

Reddy GP, Gunn M, Mitsumori LM, et al: Multislice CT and MRI of the thoracic aorta. In Webb WR, Higgins CB, editors: *Thoracic imaging: pulmonary and cardiovascular radiology*, ed 2, Philadelphia, 2010, Lippincott Williams & Wilkins.

Cross-Reference

Cardiac Imaging: The REQUISITES, ed 3, pp 377–379.

Comment

Clinical Features

The thoracic aorta is considered to be enlarged when its diameter exceeds 4 cm. Thoracic aortic enlargement is termed an aneurysm when the diameter is more than 5 cm. The maximum diameter of the aorta is an important determinant of the risk of rupture. If the diameter is 6 cm or greater, the risk of rupture in the short term is greater than 30%. Atherosclerosis is the most common cause of thoracic aortic aneurysm. Aneurysms most commonly occur in the descending aorta and aortic arch.

True and False Aneurysm

In a true aneurysm of the aorta, all three layers of the aortic wall are intact. In contrast, a false aneurysm results from a focal disruption of one or more layers of the aortic wall and may be contained by the adventitia and surrounding fibrous tissue.

Imaging

CT and MRI are the best imaging methods for evaluation of a thoracic aortic aneurysm (Figs. A-D). On CT and MRI, true aneurysms have wide necks (as in the patient in this case), and false aneurysms have narrow necks (<50% of the aneurysm diameter). True aneurysms most commonly are secondary to atherosclerosis. Other etiologies include infection, connective tissue disorders such as Marfan syndrome, aortitis, idiopathic cystic medial necrosis, complications of aortic valve disease, and aneurysm of the ductal remnant. In the imaging assessment of a thoracic aortic aneurysm, the demonstration of mural thrombus is important in patients with peripheral embolization.

Notes

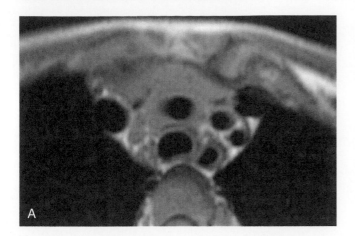

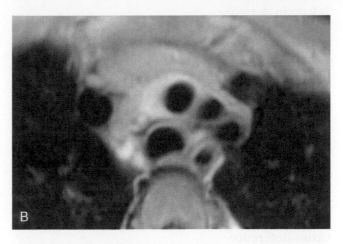

History: A patient presents with low-grade fever.

1. Which arteries are depicted in the two figures? (Choose all that apply.)
   A. Aorta
   B. Brachiocephalic artery
   C. Left common carotid artery
   D. Left subclavian artery

2. Which artery has a thickened, enhancing wall?
   A. Aorta
   B. Brachiocephalic artery
   C. Left common carotid artery
   D. Left subclavian artery

3. What is the most likely diagnosis in a young patient?
   A. Marfan syndrome
   B. Infectious arteritis
   C. Takayasu arteritis
   D. Acute hemorrhage

4. What is the most commonly involved artery in this disease?
   A. Aorta
   B. Pulmonary artery
   C. Brachiocephalic artery
   D. Subclavian artery

Takayasu Arteritis

1. B, C, and D

2. B

3. C

4. A

References

Gotway MB, Araoz PA, Macedo TA, et al: Imaging findings in Takayasu's arteritis, *AJR Am J Roentgenol* 184(6):1945-1950, 2005.

Reddy GP, Gunn M, Mitsumori LM, et al: Multislice CT and MRI of the thoracic aorta. In Webb WR, Higgins CB, editors: *Thoracic imaging: pulmonary and cardiovascular radiology*, ed 2, Philadelphia, 2010, Lippincott Williams & Wilkins.

Cross-Reference

Cardiac Imaging: The REQUISITES, ed 3, pp 393-394.

Comment

Clinical Features

Takayasu arteritis is an idiopathic disease that is characterized by wall thickening of the aorta or arch vessels, or both, and stenosis of the aorta and its branches. Other arteries, such as the pulmonary arteries, can be involved.

Imaging

In Takayasu arteritis, MRI and CT can show stenosis (Figs. A-B), occlusion, or dilation of the aorta and its branches or a combination of all three. In patients in the active phase of arteritis, gadolinium-enhanced MRI demonstrates wall thickening and enhancement of the involved vessels (Fig. B). Noninvasive imaging with MRI or CT may be particularly valuable in patients with severe stenosis or occlusion of the arch vessels or of the abdominal aorta because it may be especially difficult to pass an angiography catheter into the thoracic aorta.

Notes

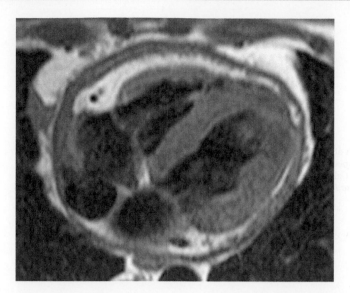

History: A patient presents with progressive dyspnea on exertion and pedal edema.

1. What etiologies can cause this finding? (Choose all that apply.)
   A. Open heart surgery
   B. Radiation therapy
   C. Viral infection
   D. Tuberculosis

2. What is the pericardial abnormality?
   A. Effusion
   B. Thickening
   C. Calcification
   D. Nodularity

3. Given the patient's symptoms, what is the most likely diagnosis?
   A. Acute pericarditis
   B. Constrictive pericarditis
   C. Tamponade
   D. Tumor

4. What is the most appropriate treatment?
   A. Antibiotics
   B. Pericardial stripping
   C. Pericardiocentesis
   D. Radiation therapy

Constrictive Pericarditis

1. A, B, C, and D

2. B

3. B

4. B

References

Wang ZJ, Reddy GP, Gotway MB, et al: CT and MR imaging of pericardial disease, *Radiographics* 23(Spec No):S167–S180, 2003.

Yared K, Baggish AL, Picard MH, et al: Multimodality imaging of pericardial diseases, *JACC Cardiovasc Imaging* 3(6):650–660, 2010.

Cross-Reference

Cardiac Imaging: The REQUISITES, ed 3, pp 269-271.

Comment

Etiology and Physiology

Constrictive pericarditis occurs when limitation in diastolic ventricular filling leads to equalization of atrial and ventricular pressure, which is known as constrictive/restrictive physiology. Patients have symptoms similar to those of congestive heart failure. Physical examination may demonstrate the classic Kussmaul sign, which is paradoxical elevation of jugular venous pressure on inspiration. Causes of constrictive pericarditis include open heart surgery, radiation therapy, uremic pericarditis, viral pericarditis, and tuberculous pericarditis (this is less common in industrialized countries).

Treatment

Constrictive pericarditis and restrictive cardiomyopathy have similar clinical presentations and findings on echocardiography and cardiac catheterization. However, it is important to differentiate between these two diseases because patients with constrictive disease usually benefit from pericardiectomy, whereas restrictive cardiomyopathy has a poor prognosis and must be managed medically or with heart transplantation.

Imaging

In the clinical setting of constrictive/restrictive physiology, pericardial thickening (≥4 mm) as demonstrated on MRI can establish the diagnosis of constrictive pericarditis (Figure). Diastolic septal dysfunction (septal bounce) on cine MRI is another key finding. Ancillary findings may be present, including dilation of the inferior vena cava, hepatic veins, and right atrium, with a narrow, tubular right ventricle. Pericardial thickening can occur in the absence of constrictive physiology. The diagnosis of constrictive pericarditis can be established only in the appropriate clinical setting of constrictive/restrictive physiology.

Notes

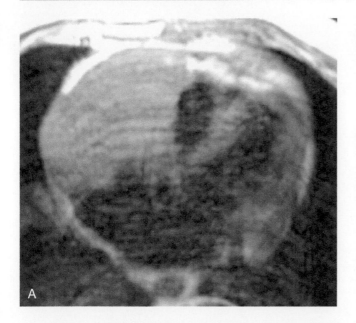

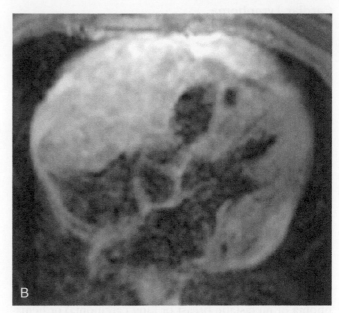

History: A patient presents with shortness of breath.

1. What should be included in the differential diagnosis? (Choose all that apply.)
   A. Metastasis
   B. Lymphoma
   C. Myxoma
   D. Angiosarcoma

2. What is the most common mass in the heart?
   A. Thrombus
   B. Myxoma
   C. Metastasis
   D. Angiosarcoma

3. Which imaging feature suggests that this mass is a tumor rather than a thrombus?
   A. Enhancement
   B. Dark signal on steady-state free precession images
   C. Size
   D. Calcification

4. Which of the following malignant features is depicted on MRI?
   A. Extension outside the heart
   B. Involvement of more than one chamber
   C. Large pericardial effusion
   D. Central necrosis

CASE 94

Cardiac Lymphoma

1. A, B, and D

2. A

3. A

4. B

Reference

Randhawa K, Ganeshan A, Hoey ET: Magnetic resonance imaging of cardiac tumors: part 2, malignant tumors and tumor-like conditions, *Curr Probl Diagn Radiol* 40(4):169-179, 2011.

Cross-Reference

Cardiac Imaging: The REQUISITES, ed 3, pp 277-278.

Comment

Etiology and Diagnosis

Approximately 98% of cardiac tumors are secondary tumors, most commonly from direct extension (lymphoma or metastatic breast or lung carcinoma) or hematogenous spread (melanoma, lung or breast carcinoma). Other primary malignant tumors are rare and include angiosarcoma, rhabdomyosarcoma, leiomyosarcoma, liposarcoma, and lymphoma. In patients with renal cell carcinoma, the tumor can enter the right atrium via the inferior vena cava. When the patient has a known malignant neoplasm elsewhere in the body, the most likely diagnosis is secondary tumor involvement of the heart. Definitive diagnosis can be made by endomyocardial or open biopsy.

Imaging

MRI shows tumor size and location as well as cardiac function. Contrast-enhanced sequences can delineate tumor margins and invasion into adjacent structures. The presence of enhancement does not signify malignancy—benign tumors also enhance. Features that suggest a primary malignant cardiac tumor include irregular or ill-defined margination, invasiveness, extension outside the heart, involvement of more than one chamber, central necrosis, large pericardial effusion, and lung nodules, which also raise the possibility of metastases. The patient in this case had non-Hodgkin lymphoma involving the mediastinum and extending into the heart (Figs. A and B).

Notes

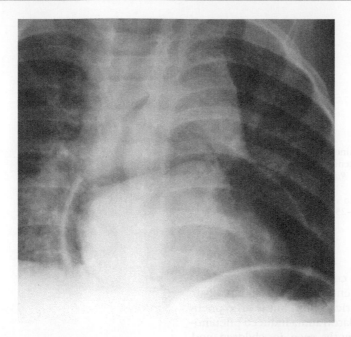

History: An intubated patient undergoes imaging.

1. What etiologies can cause this finding? (Choose all that apply.)
   A. Trauma
   B. Pericardiocentesis
   C. Barotrauma
   D. Malignant tumor

2. What is the most common cause of this finding in infants?
   A. Trauma
   B. Pericardiocentesis
   C. Barotrauma
   D. Malignant tumor

3. Which of the following is not a cause of this finding in the setting of a malignant neoplasm?
   A. Fistula with esophagus
   B. Fistula with trachea
   C. Fistula with bronchus
   D. Fistula with aorta

4. How can barotrauma result in pneumopericardium?
   A. Interstitial air dissects along the pulmonary vessels.
   B. Pneumothorax occurs and communicates with the pericardium.
   C. Pneumomediastinum occurs and communicates with the pericardium.
   D. A fistula forms between the trachea and the pericardium.

Pneumopericardium

1. A, B, C, and D

2. C

3. D

4. A

References

Katabathina VS, Restrepo CS, Martinez-Jimenez S, et al: Nonvascular, nontraumatic mediastinal emergencies in adults: a comprehensive review of imaging findings, *Radiographics* 31(4):1141–1160, 2011.

Trotman-Dickenson B: Radiology in the intensive care unit (part 2), *J Intensive Care Med* 18(5):239–252, 2003.

Comment

Etiology

Pneumopericardium is most commonly posttraumatic or iatrogenic. After pericardiocentesis, a small amount of air is frequently seen in the pericardium, but a large pneumopericardium is unusual. Barotrauma-induced pneumopericardium is most frequently seen in children and infants. In infants, barotrauma can result in a large pneumopericardium. Barotrauma causes alveolar rupture. Air dissects medially along the pulmonary vessels and bronchi towards the mediastinum. It most frequently causes pneumomediastinum but may also lead to pneumopericardium. In this setting, the pneumopericardium is usually self-limiting and resolves spontaneously. Rarely, an esophageal-pericardial fistula can develop, sometimes secondary to a malignant tumor. In this setting, patients may have a hydropneumopericardium.

Imaging

Radiography and CT can show air in the pericardial space (Figure). Tension pneumopericardium is a life-threatening condition diagnosed in the setting of hemodynamic collapse. Imaging findings on CT or MRI which suggest tamponade physiology include compression of the anterior aspect of the heart, dilated inferior vena cava, and compression or displacement of cardiac chambers. Immediate pericardial decompression is required in patients with cardiac tamponade to prevent death.

Notes

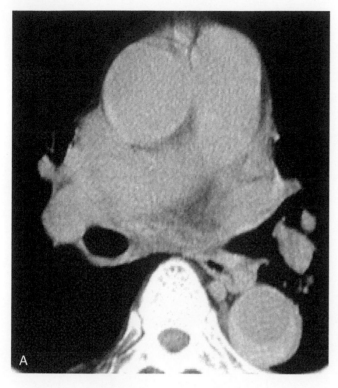

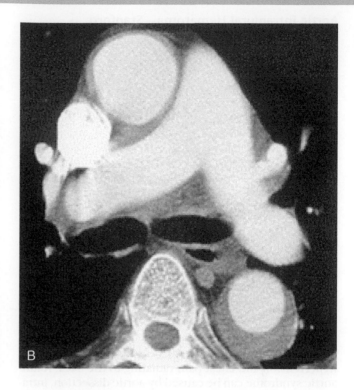

History: A patient presents with chest pain.

1. Acute aortic syndrome comprises which of the following diseases? (Choose all that apply.)
   A. Aneurysm
   B. Dissection
   C. Intramural hematoma
   D. Penetrating ulcer

2. What is the most likely diagnosis?
   A. Aneurysm
   B. Dissection
   C. Intramural hematoma
   D. Penetrating ulcer

3. What is the most likely cause of this finding?
   A. Rupture of the vasa vasorum
   B. Communication with the aortic lumen
   C. Trauma
   D. Venous bleeding

4. What is the most appropriate management of this patient?
   A. No treatment
   B. Antihypertensive medication
   C. Anticoagulation
   D. Surgery

Aortic Intramural Hematoma—Stanford Type B

1. B, C, and D

2. C

3. A

4. B

References

Chin AS, Fleischmann D: State-of-the-art computed tomography angiography of acute aortic syndrome, *Semin Ultrasound CT MR* 33(3):222–234, 2012.

Reddy GP, Gunn M, Mitsumori LM, et al: Multislice CT and MRI of the thoracic aorta. In Webb WR, Higgins CB, editors: *Thoracic imaging: pulmonary and cardiovascular radiology*, ed 2, Philadelphia, 2010, Lippincott Williams & Wilkins.

Cross-Reference

Cardiac Imaging: The REQUISITES, ed 3, p 411.

Comment

Acute Aortic Syndrome

Acute aortic syndrome is suspected in the setting of hypertension and chest pain radiating to the back. Acute aortic syndrome can be caused by aortic dissection, intramural hematoma, and penetrating aortic ulcer.

Etiology and Management

An intramural hematoma is most commonly caused by rupture of the vasa vasorum, the arteries that supply the aortic wall. The ruptured vessels bleed into the aortic wall, which can result in an intimal tear and separation of the wall—a classic dissection. If the intima does not separate, an intramural hematoma remains. The intramural hematoma may remain localized, or it can extend along the wall in an antegrade or a retrograde direction or rarely rupture through the adventitia. Intramural hematoma can be considered to be a type of dissection, and treatment is similar to a frank dissection. Stanford type B intramural hematomas are usually managed medically. Type A hematomas may need to be treated surgically, although they can be managed conservatively.

Imaging

Non–contrast-enhanced CT scan shows characteristic high-density thickening of the aortic wall, indicating intramural hematoma (Fig. A). Contrast-enhanced CT scan shows aortic wall thickening, but the high density may be difficult to appreciate (Fig. B). On MRI, the signal intensity is intermediate to high on black blood sequences. Relying solely on gadolinium-enhanced magnetic resonance angiography (MRA) can be risky in the setting of dissection because an intramural hematoma can be overlooked on this sequence.

Notes

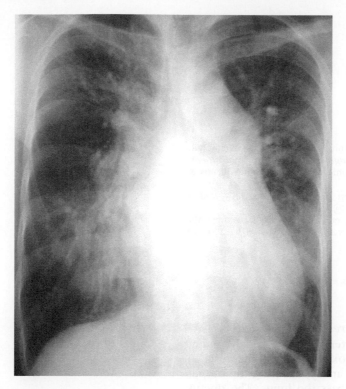

History: An acyanotic young adult presents with a cardiac murmur.

1. What should be included in the differential diagnosis? (Choose all that apply.)
   A. Atrial septal defect (ASD)
   B. Ventricular septal defect (VSD)
   C. Patent ductus arteriosus (PDA)
   D. Partial anomalous pulmonary venous connection (PAPVC)

2. What is the most likely diagnosis?
   A. ASD
   B. VSD
   C. PDA
   D. PAPVC

3. Which of these lesions commonly causes enlargement of the left atrium?
   A. PDA
   B. ASD
   C. PAPVC
   D. Pulmonary arteriovenous malformation

4. Which feature of left atrial enlargement is present in this patient's chest radiograph?
   A. Double density
   B. Splaying of the carina
   C. Prominence of the left atrial appendage
   D. Elevation of the left main bronchus

Patent Ductus Arteriosus

1. B and C

2. C

3. A

4. A

References

Higgins CB: Radiography of congenital heart disease. In Webb WR, Higgins CB, editors: *Thoracic imaging: pulmonary and cardiovascular radiology*, ed 2, Philadelphia, 2010, Lippincott Williams & Wilkins.

Kilner PJ: Imaging congenital heart disease in adults, *Br J Radiol* 84(Spec No 3):S258–S268, 2011.

Wang ZJ, Reddy GP, Gotway MB, et al: Cardiovascular shunts: MR imaging evaluation, *Radiographics* 23(Spec No):S181–S194, 2003.

Cross-Reference

Cardiac Imaging: The REQUISITES, ed 3, pp 345–349.

Comment

Embryology, Clinical Features, and Treatment

In the fetus, the ductus arteriosus is a widely patent vessel that connects the proximal descending aorta to the main or left pulmonary artery, allowing the output of the right ventricle to bypass the lungs. The ductus usually closes shortly after birth as a result of the increase in partial pressure of oxygen in the circulation. If the ductus does not close, indomethacin can be administered in the first week of life, especially in premature infants. If the ductus remains patent, pulmonary hypertension can develop. In the absence of a coexisting anomaly, the ductus should be closed by surgical ligation or by transcatheter coil embolization.

Imaging

Radiography can demonstrate increased pulmonary vascularity and enlargement of the left atrium and aortic arch (Figure). Echocardiography usually depicts the location and size of the lesion. MRI may be performed in certain patients for better delineation of the lesion or for quantification of the pulmonary-to-systemic flow ratio (Qp/Qs), which is an indicator of the severity of the shunt.

Notes

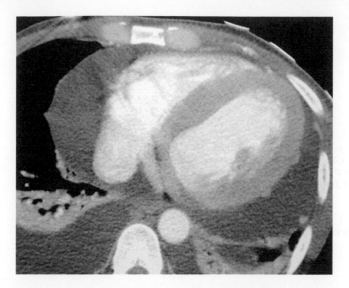

History: A patient with breast cancer undergoes imaging.

1. What should be included in the differential diagnosis? (Choose all that apply.)
   A. Metastasis
   B. Viral pericarditis
   C. Tamponade
   D. Lymphoma

2. Which of the following is most specific for a malignant effusion?
   A. High-density fluid
   B. Nodularity
   C. Thickening
   D. Enhancement

3. What is the most likely diagnosis?
   A. Metastasis
   B. Viral pericarditis
   C. Tamponade
   D. Lymphoma

4. What does pulsus paradoxus indicate?
   A. Tamponade
   B. Tumor
   C. Constriction
   D. Hemorrhage

Pericardial Metastases

1. A and D

2. B

3. A

4. A

References

Wang ZJ, Reddy GP, Gotway MB, et al: Cardiovascular shunts: MR imaging evaluation, *Radiographics* 23(Spec No):S181–S194, 2003.

Yared K, Baggish AL, Picard MH, et al: Multimodality imaging of pericardial diseases, *JACC Cardiovasc Imaging* 3(6):650–660, 2010.

Cross-Reference

Cardiac Imaging: The REQUISITES, ed 3, pp 277–278.

Comment

Pathogenesis and Etiology

Pericardial metastases are much more common than primary neoplasms of the pericardium. Tumor can seed the pericardium via lymphatic or hematogenous dissemination or invade the pericardium directly from the lung or mediastinum. Carcinomas of the breast and lung are the most common neoplasms to involve the pericardium, followed by lymphomas and melanomas.

Imaging and Diagnostic Features

Pericardial metastasis is suggested on CT or MRI by the presence of effusion with an irregularly thickened, nodular pericardium or the demonstration of a pericardial mass (Figure). The pericardial effusion may be hemorrhagic, which produces high signal intensity on spin echo MRI. Malignant disease usually enhances after the administration of contrast agent.

Notes

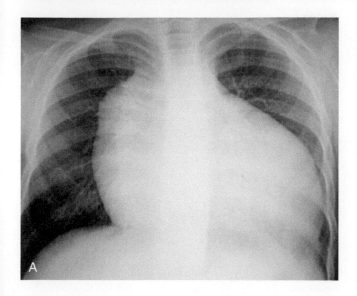

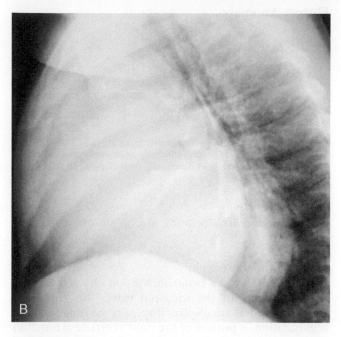

History: A patient presents with cyanosis.

1. What lesions characteristically manifest with decreased vascularity on radiography? (Choose all that apply.)
   A. Ebstein anomaly
   B. Truncus arteriosus
   C. Tetralogy of Fallot
   D. Pulmonary atresia with ventricular septal defect

2. What is the most likely diagnosis in this patient?
   A. Ebstein anomaly
   B. Truncus arteriosus
   C. Tetralogy of Fallot
   D. Pulmonary atresia with ventricular septal defect

3. Which valve is most likely abnormal?
   A. Mitral
   B. Aortic
   C. Tricuspid
   D. Pulmonary

4. Which imaging modality best assesses the valve leaflets?
   A. Echocardiography
   B. CT
   C. MRI
   D. Angiography

Ebstein Anomaly

1. A, C, and D

2. A

3. C

4. A

Reference

Higgins CB: Radiography of congenital heart disease. In Webb WR, Higgins CB, editors: *Thoracic imaging: pulmonary and cardiovascular radiology*, ed 2, Philadelphia, 2010, Lippincott Williams & Wilkins.

Cross-Reference

Cardiac Imaging: The REQUISITES, ed 3, pp 206–207.

Comment

Etiology and Physiology

Ebstein anomaly is a congenital lesion characterized by an abnormality of the tricuspid valve; the septal and posterior leaflets are displaced apically, causing tricuspid regurgitation. A portion of the right ventricle is functionally incorporated into the atrium, which is known as "atrialization of the right ventricle," although the atrialized portion of the ventricle contracts during ventricular systole. Tricuspid regurgitation causes marked enlargement of the right ventricle and atrium. Tricuspid regurgitation with a coexisting atrial septal defect results in a right-to-left shunt. Pulmonary vascularity is decreased, and cyanosis can develop. Ebstein anomaly is commonly associated with either an atrial septal defect or a patent foramen ovale. Less common associations include supraventricular tachycardia (25% to 50%), pulmonary atresia or stenosis (25%), and Wolff-Parkinson-White syndrome (10%). Maternal lithium use during the first trimester may result in Ebstein anomaly.

Imaging

Chest radiography characteristically demonstrates marked enlargement of the heart, particularly the right atrium and ventricle (Figs. A and B). Echocardiography is used for further evaluation. MRI can also be performed to assess the anatomy and to quantify the severity of regurgitation. MRI provides the same information as echocardiography and gives more reliable and reproducible information in patients with limited acoustic windows. It can assess right ventricular size and function and accurately quantitate the volume of tricuspid regurgitation, which has a direct impact on the timing of valvular surgery in these patients.

Differential Diagnosis

A few other rare conditions may manifest with cyanosis, cardiomegaly, and reduced pulmonary vascularity, including (1) severe pulmonic stenosis with a restrictive atrial septal defect, (2) tricuspid atresia with a restrictive atrial septal defect, and (3) pulmonary atresia with a restrictive ventricular septal defect.

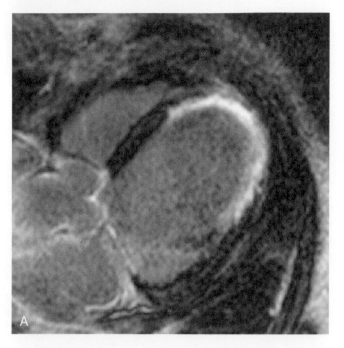

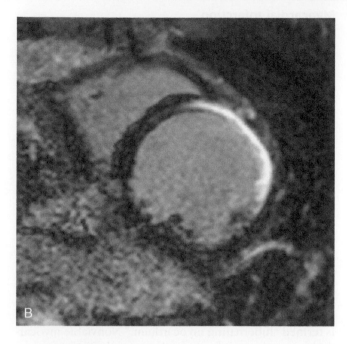

History: A patient presents with hypokinesis on echocardiography.

1. Which walls show extensive abnormality? (Choose all that apply.)
   A. Anterior
   B. Septal
   C. Lateral
   D. Apical

2. What vascular territory is involved?
   A. Left main
   B. Left anterior descending
   C. Left circumflex
   D. Right

3. What is the diagnosis?
   A. Hibernating myocardium
   B. Infarction
   C. Myocarditis
   D. Cardiomyopathy

4. What is the most appropriate management?
   A. No treatment
   B. Medical management
   C. Angioplasty and stent
   D. Coronary artery bypass graft surgery

CASE 100

Myocardial Infarction

1. A and D

2. B

3. B

4. B

Reference

Reddy GP, Pujadas S, Ordovas KG, et al: MR imaging of ischemic heart disease, *Magn Reson Imaging Clin N Am* 16(2):201–212, 2008.

Cross-Reference

Cardiac Imaging: The REQUISITES, ed 3, pp 74–76.

Comment

Clinical Issues

In a patient with impaired regional function in the left ventricle, determination of viability can be important for management decisions. In the setting of chronic poor functioning, viable but poorly functioning myocardium is termed "hibernating myocardium." Nonviable myocardium represents infarction. A revascularization procedure such as balloon angioplasty or stent or coronary artery bypass graft surgery can improve contractility in hypofunctioning but viable tissue (hibernating myocardium). However, nonviable myocardium would not benefit from a revascularization procedure.

Imaging and Implications for Management

Viability imaging with MRI is performed approximately 10 minutes after intravenous administration of gadolinium chelate contrast medium. The myocardium enhances shortly after administration of the contrast agent, but the agent washes out of viable areas. Only nonviable myocardium enhances on the delayed (10-minute) images (Figs. A and B). Revascularization would not be beneficial if the nonviable area involves more than 50% of the myocardial thickness. However, revascularization may be beneficial if the area of nonviability involves less than 50% of the myocardial thickness (e.g., if it is limited to the subendocardial region). MRI often can distinguish whether the area of nonviability involves greater than or less than 50% of the myocardial wall thickness, an advantage over positron emission tomography (PET) in the determination of viability.

Notes

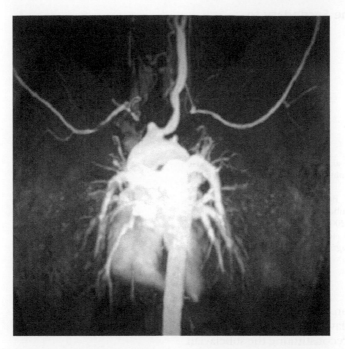

History: A 32-year-old woman presents with exercise-induced lightheadedness.

1. Which arteries are occluded? (Choose all that apply.)
   A. Aorta
   B. Brachiocephalic artery
   C. Left common carotid artery
   D. Left subclavian artery

2. Which vessel reconstitutes the occluded artery on the left?
   A. Vertebral artery
   B. Thyrocervical trunk
   C. Costocervical trunk
   D. Internal mammary artery

3. What is the most likely diagnosis?
   A. Takayasu arteritis
   B. Atherosclerosis
   C. Giant cell arteritis
   D. Marfan syndrome

4. What is the most likely cause of the patient's symptoms?
   A. Giant cell arteritis
   B. Vertebral artery occlusion
   C. Transient ischemic attack
   D. Subclavian steal syndrome

CASE 101

Subclavian Steal Syndrome Secondary to Takayasu Arteritis

1. B and D

2. A

3. A

4. D

References

Bitar R, Gladstone D, Sahlas D, et al: MR angiography of subclavian steal syndrome: pitfalls and solutions, *AJR Am J Roentgenol* 183(6):1840-1841, 2004.

Van Grimberge F, Dymarkowski S, Budts W, et al: Role of magnetic resonance in the diagnosis of subclavian steal syndrome, *J Magn Reson Imaging* 12(2):339-342, 2000.

Vummidi D, Reddy GP: Subclavian steal syndrome. In Ho VB, Reddy GP, editors: *Cardiovascular Imaging*, St Louis, 2010, Saunders.

Comment

Clinical Features

Subclavian steal phenomenon is characterized by stenosis or occlusion of the subclavian artery and reversal of flow in the vertebral artery, reconstituting the subclavian artery. Etiologies include atherosclerosis and Takayasu arteritis. Neurologic symptoms are unusual, but when they occur, the diagnosis is subclavian steal syndrome. Neurologic symptoms include lightheadedness, dizziness, upper extremity numbness, and transient ischemic attacks. Subclavian steal syndrome rarely results in stroke.

Imaging

The diagnosis can be made with Doppler ultrasound, which reveals reversal of flow in the vertebral artery. MRI and CT can show the stenotic or occluded vessels and the subclavian artery reconstitution (Figure). Phase contrast MRI and time-of-flight magnetic resonance angiography (MRA) can identify the reversal of blood flow in the vertebral artery.

Treatment

Subclavian steal phenomenon without neurologic symptoms does not require treatment, and patients generally have a benign course. Treatment of subclavian steal syndrome is aimed at fixing the subclavian artery stenosis or occlusion. At the present time, revascularization with balloon angioplasty and stent placement is the treatment of choice. Extrathoracic bypass surgery and endarterectomy are occasionally performed. Medical therapy alone is not used in the treatment of subclavian steal syndrome.

Notes

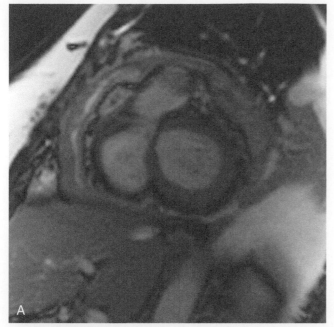

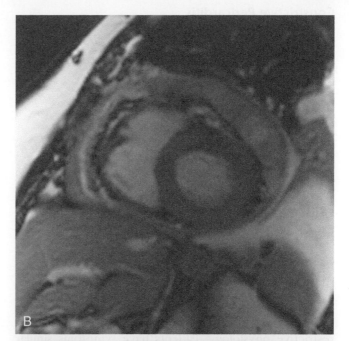

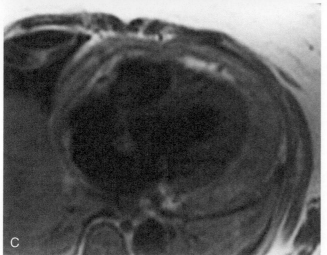

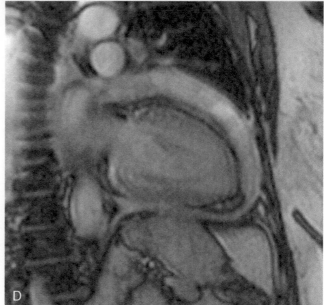

History: A patient presents with dyspnea on exertion and lower extremity edema.

1. What etiologies can cause this finding? (Choose all that apply.)
   A. Coronary artery bypass graft surgery
   B. Infection
   C. Radiation therapy
   D. Uremia

2. What is the pericardial abnormality?
   A. Effusion
   B. Thickening
   C. Calcification
   D. Nodularity

3. Given the symptoms, what is the most likely diagnosis?
   A. Acute pericarditis
   B. Constrictive pericarditis
   C. Tamponade
   D. Tumor

4. What is the most appropriate treatment?
   A. Antibiotics
   B. Pericardial stripping
   C. Pericardiocentesis
   D. Radiation therapy

CASE 102

Constrictive Pericarditis

1. A, B, C, and D

2. B

3. B

4. B

References

Wang ZJ, Reddy GP, Gotway MB, et al: CT and MR imaging of pericardial disease, *Radiographics* 23(Spec No):S167–S180, 2003.

Yared K, Baggish AL, Picard MH, et al: Multimodality imaging of pericardial diseases, *JACC Cardiovasc Imaging* 3(6):650–660, 2010.

Cross-Reference

Cardiac Imaging: The REQUISITES, ed 3, pp 269–271.

Comment

Etiology and Physiology

Constrictive pericarditis occurs when limitation in diastolic ventricular filling leads to equalization of atrial and ventricular pressures, which is known as constrictive/restrictive physiology. Patients have symptoms similar to congestive heart failure. Physical examination may demonstrate the classic Kussmaul sign, which is the paradoxical elevation of jugular venous pressure on inspiration. Causes of constrictive pericarditis include open heart surgery, radiation therapy, uremic pericarditis, viral pericarditis, and tuberculous pericarditis (less common in industrialized countries).

Treatment

Constrictive pericarditis and restrictive cardiomyopathy have similar clinical presentations and findings on echocardiography and cardiac catheterization. However, it is important to differentiate between these two diseases because patients with constrictive disease usually benefit from pericardiectomy, whereas restrictive cardiomyopathy has a poor prognosis and must be managed medically or with heart transplantation.

Imaging

In the clinical setting of constrictive/restrictive physiology, pericardial thickening (≥4 mm) as demonstrated on MRI can establish the diagnosis of constrictive pericarditis (Figs. A-D). Diastolic septal dysfunction (septal bounce) on cine MRI is another key finding. Ancillary findings may be present, including dilation of the inferior vena cava, hepatic veins, and right atrium, with a narrow, tubular right ventricle. Pericardial thickening can occur in the absence of constrictive physiology. The diagnosis of constrictive pericarditis can be established only in the appropriate clinical setting of constrictive/restrictive physiology.

Notes

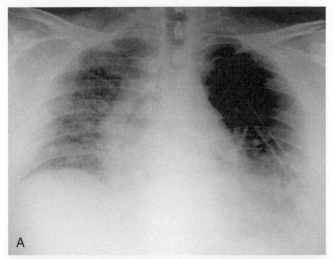

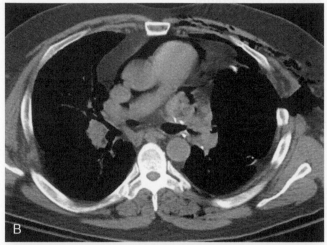

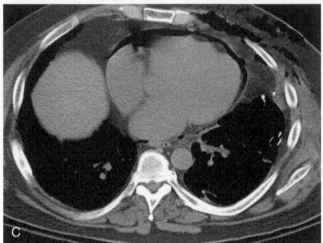

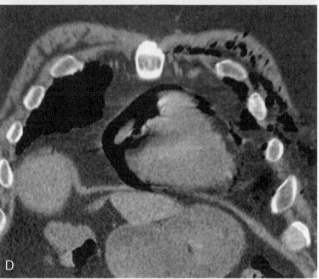

History: A patient is status post left lung transplant.

1. What etiologies can cause the cardiac finding? (Choose all that apply.)
   A. Trauma
   B. Pericardiocentesis
   C. Barotrauma
   D. Surgery

2. What is the most common cause of this finding in adults?
   A. Trauma
   B. Pericardiocentesis
   C. Barotrauma
   D. Malignant tumor

3. Which additional finding does this patient have?
   A. Subcutaneous emphysema
   B. Pneumoperitoneum
   C. Pericardial effusion
   D. Pericardial tumor

4. How can barotrauma result in pneumopericardium?
   A. Interstitial air dissects along the pulmonary vessels.
   B. Pneumoperitoneum occurs and communicates with the pericardium.
   C. Pneumothorax occurs and communicates with the pericardium.
   D. A fistula forms between the trachea and the pericardium.

Pneumopericardium

1. A, B, C, and D

2. B

3. A

4. A

Reference

Katabathina VS, Restrepo CS, Martinez-Jimenez S, et al: Nonvascular, nontraumatic mediastinal emergencies in adults: a comprehensive review of imaging findings, *Radiographics* 31(4):1141–1160, 2011.

Comment

Etiology

Pneumopericardium is most commonly posttraumatic or iatrogenic in origin. After pericardiocentesis, a small amount of air is frequently seen in the pericardium, but a large pneumopericardium is unusual. Open heart surgery is another common cause of pneumopericardium. Other thoracic surgeries are less common.

Barotrauma-induced pneumopericardium is most frequently seen in children. Although rare in adults, barotrauma can result in a large pneumopericardium. Barotrauma causes alveolar rupture. Air dissects medially along the pulmonary vessels and bronchi toward the mediastinum. It most frequently causes pneumomediastinum but may also lead to pneumopericardium. In this setting, the pneumopericardium is usually self-limiting and resolves spontaneously.

In rare instances, an esophageal-pericardial fistula can develop, sometimes secondary to a malignant tumor. In this setting, patients may have a hydropneumopericardium.

Imaging

Radiography and CT can show the air in the pericardial space (Figs. A-D). Tension pneumopericardium is a life-threatening condition that is diagnosed in the setting of hemodynamic collapse. Imaging findings on CT or MRI that suggest tamponade physiology include compression of the anterior aspect of the heart, dilated inferior vena cava, and compression or displacement of cardiac chambers. Immediate pericardial decompression is required in patients with cardiac tamponade to prevent death.

Notes

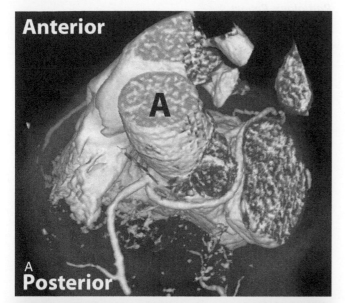

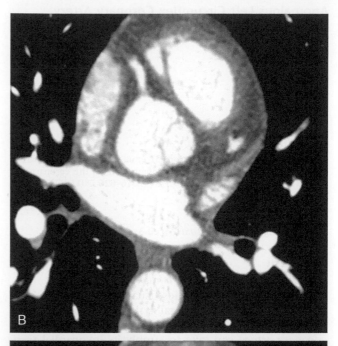

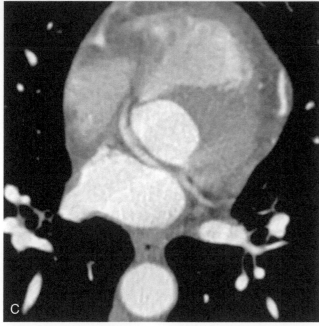

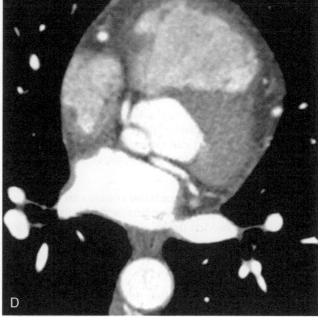

History: A young man presents with chest pain.

1. What are causes of sudden death in young adults?
   (Choose all that apply.)
   A. Marfan syndrome
   B. Anomalous coronary artery
   C. Hypertrophic cardiomyopathy
   D. Arrhythmogenic right ventricular dysplasia

2. The left main coronary artery (not shown) arises
   from the left sinus of Valsalva. Which coronary
   artery is anomalous?
   A. Left main
   B. Left anterior descending
   C. Left circumflex
   D. Right

3. What course does the anomalous vessel take?
   A. Prepulmonic
   B. Retroaortic
   C. Septal
   D. Interarterial

4. What is the usual treatment or next imaging step
   for the anomaly seen in this patient?
   A. No further evaluation
   B. Stress testing
   C. Angioplasty and stent
   D. Surgery

CASE 104

Anomalous Left Circumflex Coronary Artery with Retroaortic Course

1. A, B, C, and D

2. C

3. B

4. A

Reference

Young PM, Gerber TC, Williamson EE, et al: Cardiac imaging: part 2, normal, variant, and anomalous configurations of the coronary vasculature, *AJR Am J Roentgenol* 197(4):816–826, 2011.

Cross-Reference

Cardiac Imaging: The REQUISITES, ed 3, pp 225–228.

Comment

Anatomy and Clinical Considerations

Anomalous coronary arteries usually arise directly from the aorta. There are several types of coronary artery anomaly. There are four paths that an anomalous left coronary artery can take to supply its myocardial territory. The retroaortic and interarterial courses are the most common.

1. *Retroaortic:* An anomalous course posterior to the aorta (retroaortic) does not cause symptoms; it is considered to be a normal variant that does not need treatment (Figs. A-D).

2. *Prepulmonic:* This is also a benign variant. This vessel has an increased risk of accelerated atherosclerosis and can be injured if the patient undergoes median sternotomy, especially for repair of tetralogy of Fallot.

3. *Interarterial:* The interarterial course can lead to ischemia, with possible angina, arrhythmia, syncope, or sudden death, suggesting the need for surgical correction. Surgical options for correction include bypass graft, unroofing, or reimplantation of the anomalous artery.

4. *Septal:* This variant is often confused with the interarterial course; however, in the septal path, the artery travels through the myocardium in the proximal interventricular septum. Stress testing helps determine the clinical significance of this lesion. Patients who develop ischemia are treated surgically.

Imaging

X-ray coronary angiography can detect a coronary anomaly but often cannot definitively identify the course of the vessel. Electrocardiogram-gated CT (Figs. A-D) is used to map the course of the anomalous vessel. Charting the course of the vessel aids in management.

Radiology Report

The radiology report should address the following:

1. Origin of each coronary artery (e.g., left circumflex coronary artery arises from the right sinus of Valsalva)

2. Path the anomalous coronary artery takes to reach its myocardial territory (e.g., retroaortic, prepulmonic, septal, or interarterial)

3. Coronary artery dominance (e.g., right, left, or codominant)

4. Evidence of prior myocardial ischemia or infarction in myocardial territory supplied by anomalous coronary artery (e.g., wall thinning, subendocardial fat deposition, or wall hypokinesis if retrogated CT angiography is used)

Notes

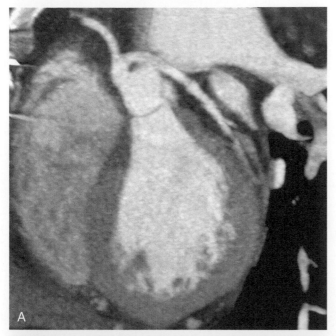

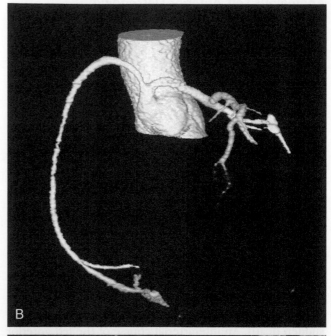

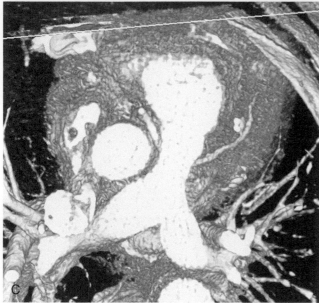

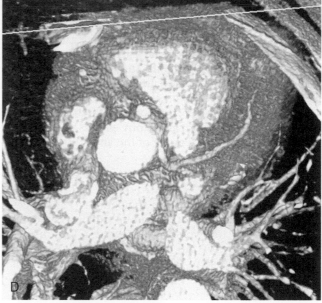

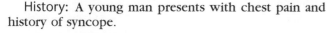

History: A young man presents with chest pain and history of syncope.

1. Which of the following are potential paths of an anomalous coronary artery? (Choose all that apply.)
   A. Retroaortic
   B. Prepulmonic
   C. Septal
   D. Interarterial

2. Which of the following best characterizes the course of the left anterior descending coronary artery?
   A. Retroaortic
   B. Prepulmonic
   C. Septal
   D. Interarterial

3. What is the most appropriate management?
   A. No treatment
   B. Beta blocker therapy
   C. Angioplasty and stent
   D. Surgery

4. What is an advantage of ECG-gated CT over coronary angiography for the evaluation of an anomalous coronary artery?
   A. Better temporal resolution
   B. Higher spatial resolution
   C. Better identification of the course of the vessel
   D. Lower radiation dose

CASE 105

Anomalous Left Anterior Descending Coronary Artery with Interarterial Course

1. A, B, C, and D

2. D

3. D

4. C

Reference

Young PM, Gerber TC, Williamson EE, et al: Cardiac imaging: part 2, normal, variant, and anomalous configurations of the coronary vasculature, *AJR Am J Roentgenol* 197(4):816–826, 2011.

Cross-Reference

Cardiac Imaging: The REQUISITES, ed 3, pp 225–228.

Comment

Clinical Features

Ectopic origin of a coronary artery is the most frequently encountered coronary artery anomaly. Certain forms are benign and are not associated with an increased risk of sudden death. An interarterial course of the left anterior descending artery, as shown in this patient, is associated with an increased risk of angina, arrhythmia, myocardial ischemia, and sudden death, and it generally requires surgical correction. Available surgical options include coronary artery bypass graft surgery, unroofing, and reimplantation of the anomalous vessel. Coronary angiography can detect an anomalous vessel but often cannot identify the course and relationship to the pulmonary artery and aorta. CT angiography guides management because it depicts the course of the anomalous vessel as well as its origin.

Imaging

Conventional x-ray coronary angiography can detect a coronary anomaly but often cannot definitively identify the course of the vessel. ECG-gated CT is used to chart the course of the anomalous vessel (Figs. A-D). Mapping the course of the vessel aids in management.

Notes

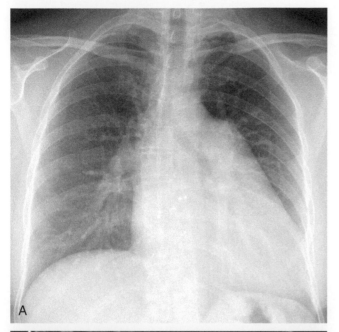

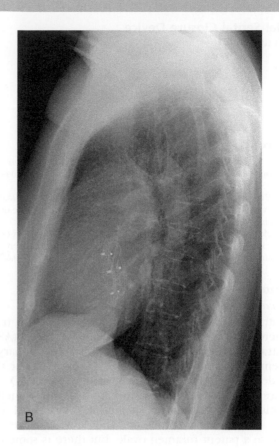

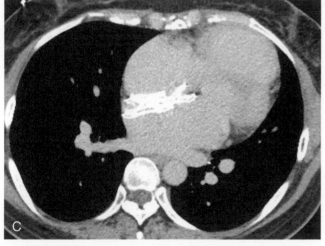

History: A 50-year-old woman presents with congenital heart disease.

1. Which lesions might have been treated with the device shown? (Choose all that apply.)
   A. Ventricular septal defect
   B. Atrial septal defect
   C. Partial anomalous pulmonary venous connection
   D. Patent foramen ovale

2. Which complication of this procedure is most readily apparent on radiographs?
   A. Unsatisfactory placement
   B. Migration
   C. Pericardial effusion
   D. Thrombus formation

3. Which of the following statements regarding limitations of the performance of cardiac MRI in this patient is true?
   A. MRI is safe to perform, and there are no limitations related to the device.
   B. MRI is safe to perform, but the device might cause an artifact.
   C. MRI is not safe to perform because of potential heating of the device.
   D. MRI is not safe to perform because of potential migration of the device.

4. Which MRI artifact would most likely be caused by the device?
   A. Aliasing
   B. Spin dephasing
   C. Ringing
   D. Susceptibility

Atrial Septal Closure Device

1. B and D

2. B

3. B

4. D

References

Burney K, Thayur N, Husain SA, et al: Imaging of implants on chest radiographs: a radiological perspective, *Clin Radiol* 62(3):204-212, 2007.

Marie Valente A, Rhodes JF: Current indications and contraindications for transcatheter atrial septal defect and patent foramen ovale device closure, *Am Heart J* 153(4 suppl):81-84, 2007.

Shellock FG: Patent ductus arteriosus (PDA), atrial septal defect (ASD), ventricular septal defect (VSD) occluders, and patent foramen ovale closure devices. MRIsafety.com (accessed February 8, 2013).

Comment

Indications and Complications

An atrial septal occluder device can be used for transcatheter closure of a secundum atrial septal defect (ASD). Contraindications include a mild shunt (pulmonary-to-systemic flow ratio <1.5:1), an ASD that is larger than the device, a defect other than a secundum ASD, and severe pulmonary hypertension. Complications include unsatisfactory placement, migration, pericardial effusion, and thrombus formation. The device can be used to close a patent foramen ovale, but there is some controversy related to this issue.

Imaging

Chest radiographs are capable of identifying the device (Figs. A and B) and assessing the possibility of migration. Other complications are more difficult to ascertain with radiographs. CT (Fig. C) can be performed to identify complications, but it has not been extensively studied for this indication. As of 2012, MRI can be performed safely, but metallic artifact can limit evaluation of the area of the device.

Notes

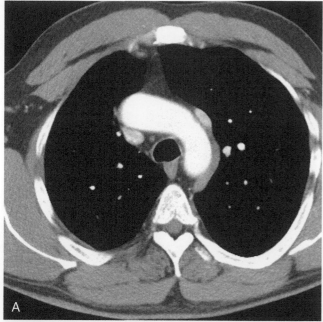

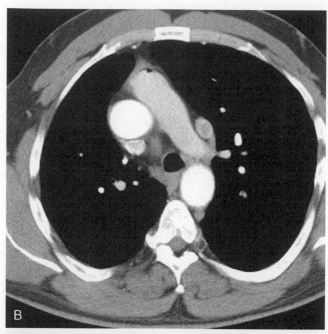

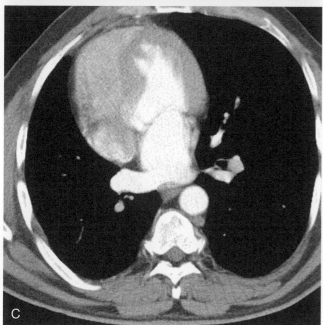

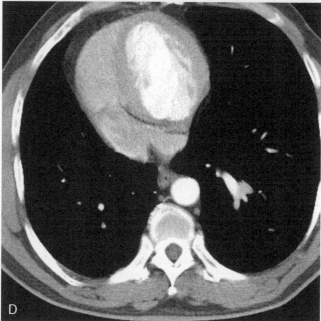

History: A patient has an abnormal cardiac silhouette.

1. What should be included in the differential diagnosis of the vessel to the left of the aortic arch in Fig. A? (Choose all that apply.)
   A. Hemiazygos vein
   B. Persistent left superior vena cava (SVC)
   C. Vertical vein
   D. Superior intercostal vein

2. Taking into account all of the figures, what is the most likely diagnosis?
   A. Hemiazygos vein
   B. Vertical vein
   C. Superior intercostal vein
   D. Persistent left SVC

3. What structure most commonly connects the right and left SVC?
   A. Coronary sinus
   B. Right brachiocephalic vein
   C. Bridging vein
   D. Right atrium

4. What other abnormality does this patient have?
   A. Dextrocardia
   B. Cardiac dextroposition
   C. Situs inversus
   D. Right aortic arch

CASE 107

Persistent Left Superior Vena Cava

1. B and C

2. D

3. C

4. B

Reference

Burney K, Young H, Barnard SA, et al: CT appearances of congenital and acquired abnormalities of the superior vena cava, *Clin Radiol* 62(9):837–842, 2007.

Cross-Reference

Cardiac Imaging: The REQUISITES, ed 3, pp 27–29.

Comment

Etiology

Persistent left SVC results when the left anterior cardinal vein persists after birth. The left brachiocephalic vein drains into the left SVC, which usually connects to the coronary sinus. The coronary sinus may be dilated from the increase in flow, especially if there is no right SVC. Most individuals are asymptomatic, and their anatomy is otherwise normal. Most individuals with a persistent left SVC have a right SVC as well—hence the designation "duplicated SVC."

Associated Anomalies

Rarely, the left SVC drains into the left atrium. In this situation, multiple severe cardiac anomalies may coexist, such as common atrium, atrioventricular canal defect, single ventricle, asplenia, and polysplenia. Persistent left SVC is also associated with atrial septal defect, tetralogy of Fallot, and partial and total anomalous pulmonary venous connection.

Imaging

Persistent left SVC may be identified on a chest radiograph after placement of a central venous catheter, pulmonary artery catheter, or pacemaker. The anomaly may be seen incidentally on a CT scan or MRI, which can demonstrate a round or oval vessel to the left of the aortic arch (Fig. A) and drainage into the coronary sinus (Figs. B-D).

Notes

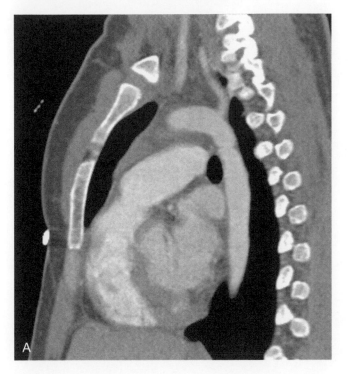

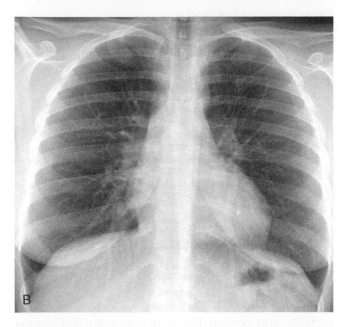

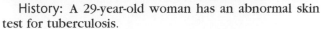

History: A 29-year-old woman has an abnormal skin test for tuberculosis.

1. What should be included in the differential diagnosis? (Choose all that apply.)
   A. Coarctation
   B. Pseudocoarctation
   C. Double aortic arch
   D. Right aortic arch

2. The patient's blood pressure is unknown. If the patient has normal systemic blood pressure, what is the most likely diagnosis, based on the radiograph?
   A. Coarctation
   B. Pseudocoarctation
   C. Double aortic arch
   D. Right aortic arch

3. Based on the CT image, what is the most likely diagnosis?
   A. Coarctation
   B. Pseudocoarctation
   C. Double aortic arch
   D. Right aortic arch

4. What is an advantage of CT over MRI for evaluation of coarctation of the aorta?
   A. It is safer in patients with renal insufficiency.
   B. It can determine functional significance.
   C. It provides better spatial resolution.
   D. CT has a lower radiation dose than MRI.

CASE 108

Coarctation of the Aorta

1. A and B

2. B

3. A

4. C

References

Hom JJ, Ordovas K, Reddy GP: Velocity-encoded cine MR imaging in aortic coarctation: functional assessment of hemodynamic events, *Radiographics* 28(2):407-416, 2008.

Kilner PJ: Imaging congenital heart disease in adults, *Br J Radiol* 84(Spec No 3):S258-S268, 2011.

Cross-Reference

Cardiac Imaging: The REQUISITES, ed 3, pp 72, 160-162, 420.

Comment

Clinical Features

Congenital coarctation is most commonly discrete and juxtaductal in location (Fig. A). Hypertension is a common finding, often localized to the upper extremities.

Imaging

Radiographs may be nonspecific, but they can show an abnormal aortic knob (Fig. B), a "figure 3" contour of the proximal descending aorta, and rib notching. Rib notching occurs as a result of dilated intercostal arteries, which function as a collateral route for blood flow around the site of aortic narrowing. The main pathway of collateral flow proceeds as follows: aortic arch to subclavian artery to internal mammary artery to intercostal artery to descending thoracic aorta. Additional collateral pathways around the coarctation include the thyrocervical, thoracoacromial trunk, and epigastric arteries. Echocardiography can demonstrate the pressure gradient across the stenosis. CT and MRI can be used to delineate the anatomy. CT has the disadvantage of ionizing radiation, and MRI has the ability to determine the hemodynamic significance of the coarctation. Another benefit of MRI over CT and other modalities is its ability to distinguish pseudocoarctation from aortic coarctation. MRI determines functional information by measuring the pressure gradient across the narrowing and by determining the volume of collateral flow through the use of velocity-encoded cine phase contrast MRI. Aortic pseudocoarctation does not have a pressure gradient or collateral flow.

Associations

The most common association with coarctation is a bicuspid aortic valve followed by Turner syndrome. Aortic coarctation is frequently fatal if it is left untreated. Causes of death include congestive heart failure, aortic dissection, endocarditis, and aortic rupture. Patients are also predisposed to cerebral aneurysms with intracranial hemorrhage secondary to carotid artery hypertension.

Notes

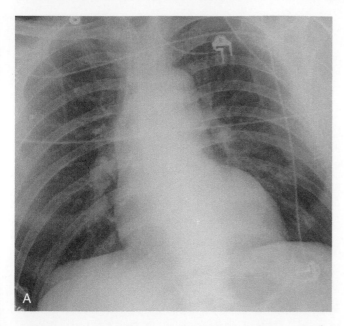

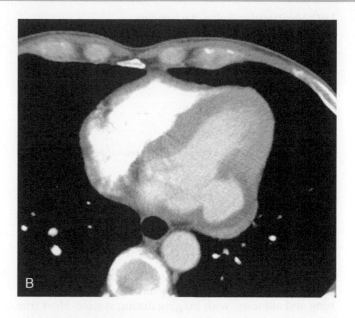

History: A patient presents with congestive heart failure.

1. What should be included in the differential diagnosis for the cardiac contour abnormality based on the radiograph? (Choose all that apply.)
   A. Mitral stenosis
   B. Pericardial cyst
   C. Ventricular aneurysm
   D. Metastasis

2. Based on the CT image, what is the most likely diagnosis?
   A. Mitral stenosis
   B. Pericardial cyst
   C. Ventricular aneurysm
   D. Metastasis

3. Which of the following features is most specific for the CT diagnosis of a false aneurysm?
   A. Narrow ostium
   B. Inferodiaphragmatic location
   C. Large size
   D. Disruption of the ventricular wall

4. What is the most appropriate management of a false aneurysm?
   A. No therapy
   B. Medical management
   C. Stent graft
   D. Surgery

Left Ventricular False Aneurysm
1. B, C, and D

2. C

3. A

4. D

Reference
White RD: MR and CT assessment for ischemic cardiac disease, *J Magn Reson Imaging* 19(6):659-675, 2004.⑨

Cross-Reference
Cardiac Imaging: The REQUISITES, ed 3, pp 236-237.

Comment
Pathology and Etiology

Left ventricular aneurysms result from a transmural myocardial infarction. True aneurysms have focal wall thinning and akinesis, with bulging during systole. Most true aneurysms are located in the anteroapical region of the left ventricle and have wide necks. A false aneurysm represents a contained rupture. Most false aneurysms are inferoposterior in location and are connected to the left ventricle via a narrow neck (Fig. B).

Treatment

True aneurysms are usually managed medically, unless there is substantial dysfunction, such as heart failure, arrhythmia, or peripheral embolization of thrombus. False aneurysms are usually resected because of the high risk of rupture.

Imaging and Diagnostic Criteria

With MRI or CT, true and false aneurysms can be differentiated on the basis of their necks. Location is suggestive but not definitive for differentiating a true aneurysm from a false aneurysm. The inferoposterior location of the aneurysm and the narrow neck (<50% of the diameter of the aneurysm) indicate a false aneurysm (Figs. A and B).

Notes

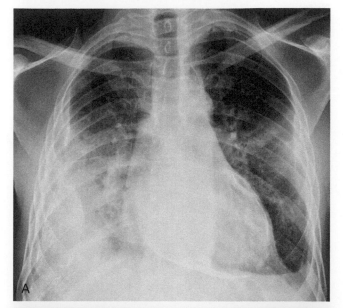

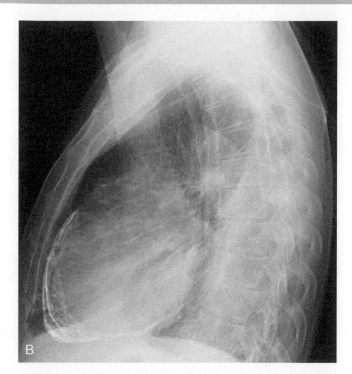

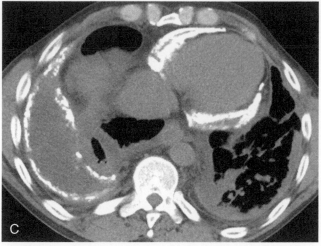

History: A patient presents with dyspnea on exertion.

1. What etiologies can cause the cardiac finding? (Choose all that apply.)
   A. Tuberculosis
   B. Uremia
   C. Mesothelioma
   D. Hemorrhage

2. Which cardiac structure is calcified?
   A. Left ventricle
   B. Pericardium
   C. Valve
   D. Coronary artery

3. Given the patient's clinical presentation, what is the most likely diagnosis?
   A. Tumor
   B. Tamponade
   C. Acute pericarditis
   D. Constrictive pericarditis

4. Given the other findings in the chest, what is the most likely etiology of the cardiac abnormality?
   A. Tuberculosis
   B. Uremia
   C. Mesothelioma
   D. Hemorrhage

CASE 110

Calcific Pericarditis

1. A, B, and D

2. B

3. D

4. A

References

Gowda RM, Boxt LM: Calcifications of the heart, *Radiol Clin North Am* 42(3):603–617, 2004.

Walker CM, Reddy GP, Steiner RM: Radiology of the heart. In Rosendorff C, editor: *Essential Cardiology*, ed 3, Boston, 2012, Saunders.

Cross-Reference

Cardiac Imaging: The REQUISITES, ed 3, pp 10, 79–82.

Comment

Calcific Pericarditis

Chronic pericarditis can follow uremic pericarditis, viral or tuberculous infection, radiation therapy, or open heart surgery. In chronic pericarditis, pericardial calcification most often results from tuberculosis. Because tuberculous pericarditis is rare in industrialized countries, pericardial calcification (Figs. A-C) occurs in less than 20% of patients with chronic pericarditis. Calcific pericarditis does not necessarily cause symptoms of constriction.

Constrictive Pericarditis

In the setting of chronic pericarditis, a patient may have constrictive pericarditis. Constrictive pericarditis is difficult to distinguish from restrictive cardiomyopathy. If a patient has constrictive/restrictive physiology, characterized by dyspnea, lower extremity edema, pleural effusions, and ascites, imaging studies can be used to differentiate constrictive pericarditis from restrictive cardiomyopathy. This differentiation is important because treatments are vastly different. Constrictive pericarditis is treated surgically with pericardial stripping, whereas restrictive cardiomyopathy is managed medically or with heart transplantation. Pericardial thickening of at least 4 mm (best seen on MRI or CT), pericardial calcification (Figs. A-C), and abnormal diastolic septal motion ("septal bounce") help establish the diagnosis of constrictive pericarditis.

Restrictive Cardiomyopathy

Patients with restrictive cardiomyopathy and patients with constrictive pericarditis have similar symptoms. On imaging, the pericardial thickness and systolic function are generally normal. Symptoms are due to diastolic dysfunction leading to restricted ventricular filling and reduced cardiac output. Inversion recovery late gadolinium enhancement imaging is helpful in suggesting a specific diagnosis. Causes of restrictive cardiomyopathy include amyloidosis, radiation therapy, sarcoidosis, and hemochromatosis.

Notes

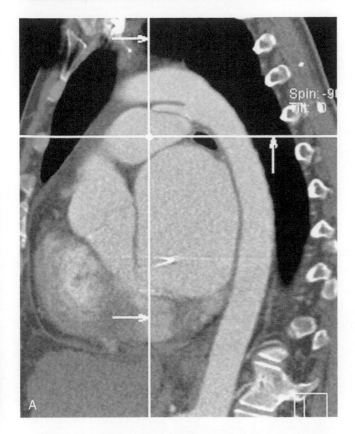

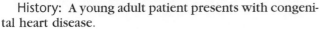

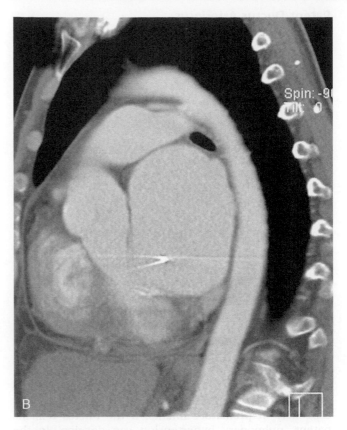

History: A young adult patient presents with congenital heart disease.

1. Which of the following are advantages of MRI over CT for the evaluation of congenital heart disease? (Choose all that apply.)
   A. MRI is safer in patients with renal insufficiency.
   B. MRI can determine function.
   C. MRI provides better spatial resolution.
   D. MRI has a lower radiation dose.

2. What is the most likely diagnosis?
   A. Aortic arch anomaly or vascular ring
   B. Coarctation of the aorta
   C. Patent ductus arteriosus
   D. Pulmonary sling

3. In infancy, which of the following symptoms or complications is least likely?
   A. Congestive heart failure
   B. Murmur
   C. Shortness of breath
   D. Cyanosis

4. Which of the following is not an appropriate treatment in this patient?
   A. Intravenous indomethacin or ibuprofen
   B. Coil embolization
   C. Transcatheter occlusion device
   D. Surgical ligation

Patent Ductus Arteriosus

1. A, B, and D

2. C

3. D

4. A

References

Kilner PJ: Imaging congenital heart disease in adults, *Br J Radiol* 84(Spec No 3):S258–S268, 2011.

Wang ZJ, Reddy GP, Gotway MB, et al: Cardiovascular shunts: MR imaging evaluation, *Radiographics* 23(Spec No):S181–S194, 2003.

Cross-Reference

Cardiac Imaging: The REQUISITES, ed 3, pp 345–349.

Comment

Embryology, Clinical Features, and Treatment

In the fetus, the ductus arteriosus is a widely patent vessel that connects the proximal descending aorta to the main or left pulmonary artery, allowing the output of the right ventricle to bypass the lungs. The ductus usually closes shortly after birth as a result of the increase in the partial pressure of oxygen in the circulation. If the ductus does not close, intravenous indomethacin or ibuprofen can be administered in the first week of life, especially in premature infants. If the ductus remains patent, pulmonary hypertension can develop. In the absence of a coexisting anomaly, the ductus should be closed by surgical ligation or by transcatheter coil embolization or occluder device.

Imaging

Radiography can demonstrate increased pulmonary vascularity and enlargement of the left atrium and aortic arch. Echocardiography usually depicts the location and size of the lesion. MRI or CT may be performed in certain patients for better delineation of the lesion (Figs. A and B), and velocity-encoded cine phase contrast MRI can be performed for quantification of the pulmonary-to-systemic flow ratio, which is an indicator of the severity of the shunt.

Notes

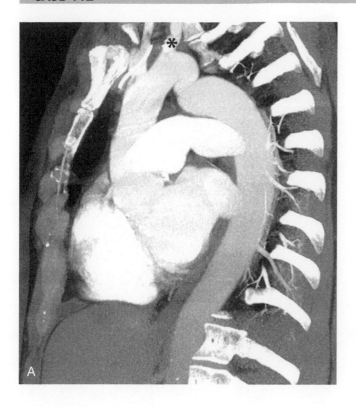

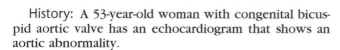

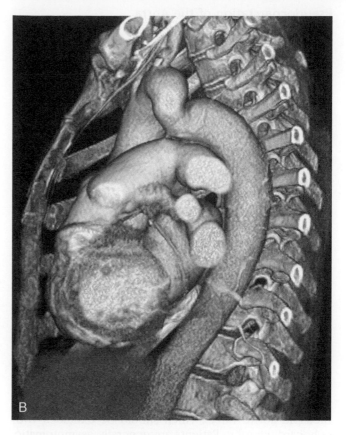

History: A 53-year-old woman with congenital bicuspid aortic valve has an echocardiogram that shows an aortic abnormality.

1. What are advantages of CT over MRI for evaluation of the thoracic aorta? (Choose all that apply.)
   A. No need for electrocardiogram (ECG) gating
   B. No need for gadolinium-based contrast agent
   C. Better spatial resolution
   D. Faster imaging time

2. Which of the following is present in pseudocoarctation?
   A. Kinking of the aorta
   B. Hemodynamically significant narrowing
   C. Collateral blood flow
   D. Rib notching

3. What is the most likely diagnosis?
   A. Coarctation
   B. Pseudocoarctation
   C. Double aortic arch
   D. Right aortic arch

4. In Fig. A, what structure is indicated by the asterisk?
   A. Left common carotid artery
   B. Left subclavian artery
   C. Left vertebral artery
   D. Innominate (brachiocephalic artery)

Pseudocoarctation of the Aorta

1. C and D

2. A

3. B

4. B

References

Reddy GP, Gunn M, Mitsumori LM, et al: Multislice CT and MRI of the thoracic aorta. In Webb WR, Higgins CB, editors: *Thoracic imaging: pulmonary and cardiovascular radiology*, ed 2, Philadelphia, 2010, Lippincott Williams & Wilkins.

Sebastia C, Quiroga S, Boye R, et al: Aortic stenosis: spectrum of diseases depicted at multisection CT, *Radiographics* 23(Spec No):S79–S91, 2003.

Cross-Reference

Cardiac Imaging: The REQUISITES, ed 3, pp 424–427.

Comment

Etiology and Anatomy

Pseudocoarctation is an uncommon congenital anomaly caused by elongation of the aortic arch and kinking or buckling at the site of attachment to the ligamentum arteriosum. There is no narrowing of the vessel lumen, and there is no hemodynamic gradient. Similar to aortic coarctation, there is an association with a congenitally bicuspid aortic valve, which should be excluded with echocardiography. Patients are generally asymptomatic, and the anomaly is discovered on imaging performed for other reasons. No treatment is necessary in most cases.

Imaging

Radiographs are often nonspecific, but they can show an abnormal aortic knob and a "figure 3" contour of the proximal descending aorta. On CT and MRI, the appearance of the aorta in pseudocoarctation is similar to aorta in true coarctation (Figs. A and B). CT has the disadvantage of ionizing radiation, and MRI may be better at distinguishing pseudocoarctation from aortic coarctation. MRI determines functional information by measuring the pressure gradient across the narrowing and by determining the volume of collateral flow through the use of velocity-encoded cine phase contrast MRI. In pseudocoarctation, there is no narrowing of the vessel lumen and no pressure gradient across the site of kinking. Collateral circulation does not develop, and rib notching does not occur. Thoracic aortic aneurysms occasionally develop around the pseudocoarctation, and these should be monitored closely and treated.

Notes

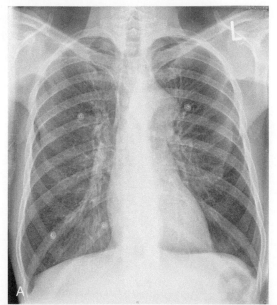

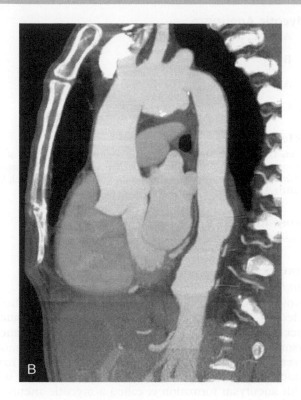

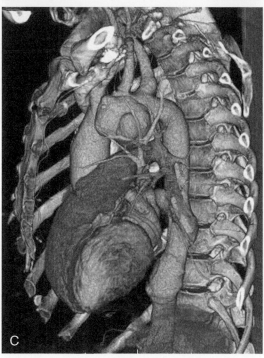

History: A 33-year-old man presents with *Staphylococcus aureus* bacteremia.

1. What are potential etiologies of the abnormality seen on the frontal radiograph? (Choose all that apply.)
   A. Lymphoma
   B. Lung cancer
   C. Reactive lymphadenopathy
   D. Aortic aneurysm

2. Based on the CT scan, which portion of the aorta is most abnormal?
   A. Ascending
   B. Arch
   C. Descending
   D. Abdominal

3. What is the most likely diagnosis of the arch abnormality?
   A. True aneurysm
   B. Pseudoaneurysm
   C. Aortic diverticulum
   D. Intramural hematoma

4. What is the most likely etiology?
   A. Trauma
   B. Atherosclerosis
   C. Infection
   D. Marfan syndrome

CASE 113

Mycotic Aneurysm

1. A, B, C, and D

2. B

3. A

4. C

Reference

Reddy GP, Gunn M, Mitsumori LM, et al: Multislice CT and MRI of the thoracic aorta. In Webb WR, Higgins CB, editors: *Thoracic imaging: pulmonary and cardiovascular radiology*, ed 2, Philadelphia, 2010, Lippincott Williams & Wilkins.

Cross-Reference

Cardiac Imaging: The REQUISITES, ed 3, pp 377-379, 398.

Comment

Etiology and Pathology

Etiologies of an aortic pseudoaneurysm include atherosclerosis (penetrating aortic ulcer), infection, trauma (deceleration injury), and iatrogenic injury. Pseudoaneurysms are characterized by disruption of one or more layers of the vessel wall, whereas true aneurysms have intact walls. A nonsyphilitic infection of the aortic wall with aneurysm formation is called a mycotic aneurysm and is most commonly seen in patients with aortic wall damage (i.e., in a setting of trauma, endocarditis, or drug abuse). Pathogens most commonly responsible for mycotic aneurysms include *Streptococcus, Staphylococcus, Pneumococcus,* and *Salmonella* species. *Mycobacterium tuberculosis* can affect the aorta by contiguous spread from infected lymph nodes or the spine.

True and False Aneurysm

In a true aneurysm of the aorta, all three layers of the aortic wall are intact. In contrast, a false aneurysm results from a focal disruption of one or more layers of the aortic wall and may be contained by the adventitia and surrounding fibrous tissue.

Imaging

CT and MRI are the best imaging methods for evaluation of a thoracic aortic aneurysm. Disruption of the wall is difficult to identify by imaging examination. However, many observers use a rule of thumb: a relatively narrow ostium (<50% of the aneurysm diameter) suggests that the outpouching is a pseudoaneurysm, and a wide ostium suggests a true aneurysm. Most mycotic aneurysms have a saccular configuration, may contain peripheral thrombus, and can grow rapidly. There may be periaortic fat infiltration from associated inflammation. The case shown is atypical for mycotic aneurysm because the saccular outpouching has a relatively wide neck (Figs. A-C).

Notes

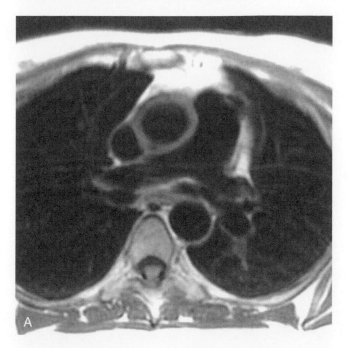

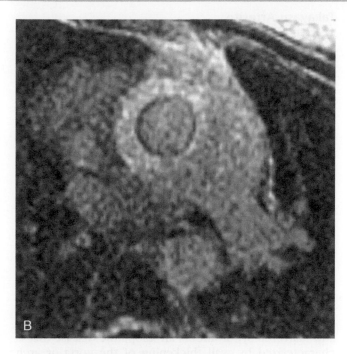

History: A 51-year-old woman presents with chest pain and an elevated erythrocyte sedimentation rate.

1. What should be included in the differential diagnosis? (Choose all that apply.)
   A. Intramural hematoma
   B. Atherosclerosis
   C. Acute traumatic injury
   D. Takayasu arteritis

2. Which artery has a thickened, enhancing wall?
   A. Ascending aorta
   B. Descending aorta
   C. Main pulmonary artery
   D. Left pulmonary artery

3. What is the most likely diagnosis?
   A. Intramural hematoma
   B. Takayasu arteritis
   C. Marfan syndrome
   D. Infectious arteritis

4. What artery is most commonly involved in this disease?
   A. Aorta
   B. Pulmonary artery
   C. Brachiocephalic artery
   D. Subclavian artery

Takayasu Arteritis

1. A and D

2. A

3. B

4. A

References

Gotway MB, Araoz PA, Macedo TA, et al: Imaging findings in Takayasu's arteritis, *AJR Am J Roentgenol* 184(6):1945-1950, 2005.

Reddy GP, Gunn M, Mitsumori LM, et al: Multislice CT and MRI of the thoracic aorta. In Webb WR, Higgins CB, editors: *Thoracic imaging: pulmonary and cardiovascular radiology*, ed 2, Philadelphia, 2010, Lippincott Williams & Wilkins.

Cross-Reference

Cardiac Imaging: The REQUISITES, ed 3, pp 393-394.

Comment

Clinical Features

Takayasu arteritis (synonyms include pulseless disease and Martorell syndrome) is an idiopathic disease that is characterized by wall thickening of the aorta or arch vessels (or both) with stenosis of the aorta and its branches. Other arteries, such as the pulmonary arteries, can be involved. The two main large vessel arteritides include Takayasu arteritis and giant cell arteritis. Takayasu arteritis most commonly affects Asian women 10 to 40 years of age, whereas giant cell arteritis occurs in patients older than 50. The treatment of choice generally is high-dose corticosteroids.

Imaging

In Takayasu arteritis, MRI and CT can show stenosis, occlusion, or dilation of the aorta and its branches, or a combination of all three. In patients in the active phase of arteritis, gadolinium-enhanced MRI demonstrates wall thickening and enhancement of the involved vessels (Figs. A and B). Noninvasive imaging with MRI or CT may be particularly valuable in patients with severe stenosis or occlusion of the arch vessels or of the abdominal aorta because it may be especially difficult to pass an angiography catheter into the thoracic aorta. An aortic wall thickness of greater than 3 mm has been proposed as a marker for early Takayasu arteritis. Concentric aortic wall calcification has been described in patients with late-stage Takayasu arteritis. Positron emission tomography (PET) is useful for monitoring disease response in patients with large vessel vasculitides. Decreasing fluorodeoxyglucose (FDG) activity is considered a favorable response to therapy and may be seen before decreased aortic wall thickening is shown on anatomic imaging.

Notes

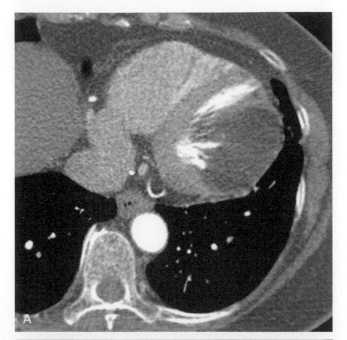

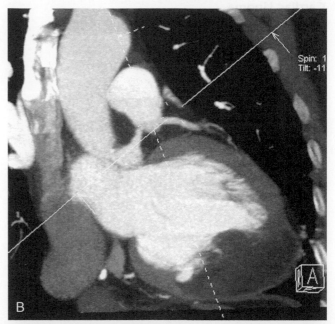

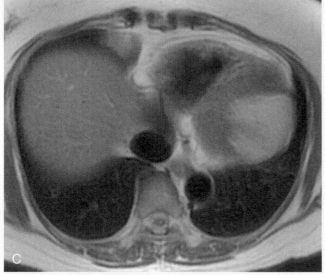

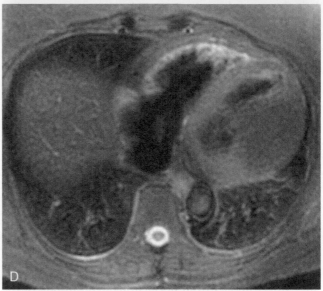

History: A 64-year-old woman presents with chest pain.

1. What should be included in the differential diagnosis? (Choose all that apply.)
   A. Cyst
   B. Hematoma
   C. Lipoma
   D. Metastasis

2. What is the most likely location of the mass?
   A. Pericardium
   B. Myocardium
   C. Left atrium
   D. Right atrium

3. What is the most likely diagnosis?
   A. Cyst
   B. Hematoma
   C. Lipoma
   D. Metastasis

4. What is the most appropriate management?
   A. No treatment
   B. Chemotherapy
   C. Radiation therapy
   D. Surgery

CASE 115

Cardiac Lipoma

1. C and D

2. B

3. C

4. D

References

Hoey ET, Mankad K, Puppala S, et al: MRI and CT appearances of cardiac tumours in adults, *Clin Radiol* 64(12):1214-1230, 2009.

O'Donnell DH, Abbara S, Chaithiraphan V, et al: Cardiac tumors: optimal cardiac MR sequences and spectrum of imaging appearances, *AJR Am J Roentgenol* 193(2):377-387, 2009.

Cross-Reference

Cardiac Imaging: The REQUISITES, ed 3, p 281.

Comment

Clinical Features

Cardiac lipoma is an uncommon benign encapsulated tumor that most commonly occurs in the right atrium. It is the second most common benign primary cardiac neoplasm after myxoma. Other locations include the epicardium, endocardium, interatrial septum, and left ventricle. Lipomas may grow into the pericardial space when they arise from the epicardium or into a ventricular chamber when they arise from the endocardium. Lipomas tend to be soft and flexible, and even large tumors may not compress the heart. Patients are usually asymptomatic. If there are symptoms of compression, such as pain or shortness of breath, surgical resection is usually performed.

Imaging Features

On CT, a cardiac lipoma manifests as a homogeneous, low-density mass with negative Hounsfield units (Figs. A and B). There is generally no enhancement, and there are no signs of invasion. MRI sequences with and without fat saturation can be used to show that the mass is composed of fat (Figs. C and D). It is important to differentiate cardiac lipoma from lipomatous hypertrophy of the interatrial septum, which has a bilobed appearance and is unencapsulated. Cardiac lipoma does not have significant fluorodeoxyglucose (FDG) uptake, whereas lipomatous hypertrophy may be FDG avid from associated brown fat.

Associations

Multiple fat-containing masses within myocardium have been described in patients with tuberous sclerosis. Current pathologic literature suggests these fatty lesions may represent unencapsulated fat cells rather than true encapsulated cardiac lipomas.

Notes

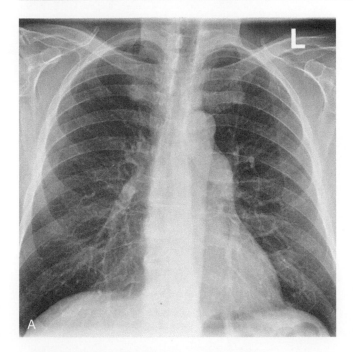

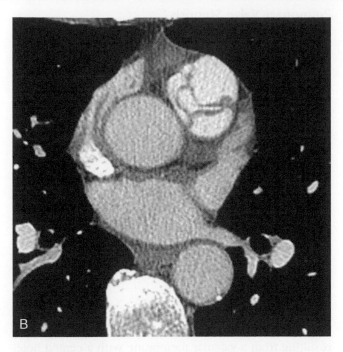

History: A patient presents with malaise.

1. What imaging study can be performed to evaluate the abnormality seen on the radiograph? (Choose all that apply.)
   A. Echocardiography
   B. CT
   C. MRI
   D. Stress perfusion scintigraphy

2. What is the most likely diagnosis?
   A. Mitral stenosis
   B. Mitral regurgitation
   C. Pulmonary stenosis
   D. Pulmonary regurgitation

3. What is the most common cause of pulmonary stenosis?
   A. Trauma
   B. Congenital
   C. Rheumatic heart disease
   D. Carcinoid syndrome

4. What is the most common intervention for treatment of this lesion?
   A. Balloon valvuloplasty
   B. Stent placement
   C. Transcatheter valve replacement
   D. Surgical valve replacement

Pulmonary Valve Stenosis

1. A, B, and C

2. C

3. B

4. A

References

Kenny D, Hijazi ZM: State-of-the-art percutaneous pulmonary valve therapy, *Expert Rev Cardiovasc Ther* 10(5):589–597, 2012.

Kilner PJ: Imaging congenital heart disease in adults, *Br J Radiol* 84(Spec No):S258–S268, 2011.

Walker CM, Reddy GP, Steiner RM: Radiology of the heart. In Rosendorff C, editor: *Essential Cardiology*, ed 3, Philadelphia, 2012, Saunders.

Cross-Reference

Cardiac Imaging: The REQUISITES, ed 3, pp 195–202.

Comment

Etiology and Clinical Considerations

Pulmonary valve stenosis is most commonly congenital, resulting from a valvular membrane with a central hole, a bicuspid valve, or valve dysplasia (associated with Noonan syndrome). Acquired causes include carcinoid and rheumatic heart disease.

Treatment

Balloon valvuloplasty is the most common intervention used to treat this lesion. Infants and young children are often treated with balloon valvuloplasty. One complication of balloon valvuloplasty is pulmonary regurgitation. Older children and adults usually require valve replacement.

Radiography

Chest radiographic findings vary depending on patient age and associated abnormalities. In infants, a large thymus may obscure the central pulmonary arteries, and the only sign of disease may be decreased pulmonary flow. In older children and adults, there is poststenotic dilation of the main pulmonary artery (Fig. A) and often of the left pulmonary artery. The right pulmonary artery is normal. Cardiac size is usually normal, unless the stenosis is severe enough to obstruct cardiac output.

Further Imaging

Echocardiography demonstrates thickening and poor excursion of the valve leaflets and a jet across the lesion. CT and MRI can also show leaflet thickening (Fig. B) and limitation of excursion. Angiography demonstrates doming, thickening, and poor excursion of the valve leaflets. A jet of contrast agent can be seen passing across the valve.

Notes

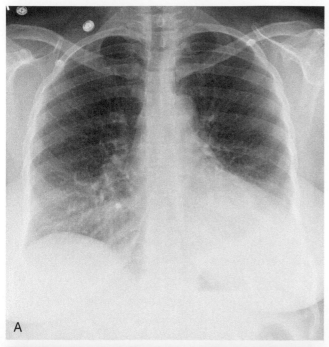

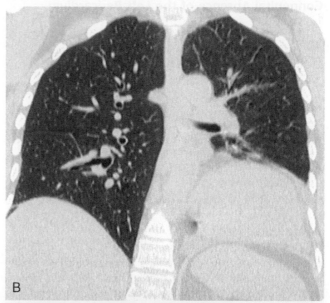

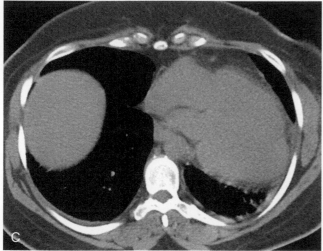

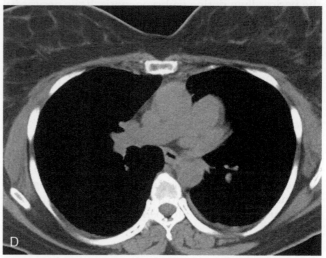

History: A patient scheduled to undergo knee surgery presents for preoperative evaluation.

1. Which findings are present? (Choose all that apply.)
   A. Rotation of the heart
   B. Cardiomegaly
   C. Deviation of trachea and esophagus
   D. Lung between the aorta and pulmonary artery

2. Which structure is bulging along the left heart border?
   A. Aorta
   B. Pulmonary artery
   C. Left atrial appendage
   D. Left ventricle

3. What is the most likely diagnosis?
   A. Absence of the pericardium
   B. Hypoplastic lung
   C. Mitral stenosis
   D. Mitral regurgitation

4. What is the most appropriate management?
   A. No further evaluation or treatment
   B. Echocardiography
   C. Cardiac catheterization
   D. Surgery

CASE 117

Congenital Absence of the Left Pericardium

1. A and D

2. C

3. A

4. A

Reference

Wang ZJ, Reddy GP, Gotway MB, et al: CT and MR imaging of pericardial disease, *Radiographics* 23(Spec No):S167–S180, 2003.

Cross-Reference

Cardiac Imaging: The REQUISITES, ed 3, p 78.

Comment

Clinical Features

Congenital absence of the left pericardium is usually asymptomatic and needs no treatment. It is thought to occur secondary to a compromise of vascular supply to the pericardium during embryogenesis. If the pericardial defect is small and the left atrium, atrial appendage, or left ventricle herniates through it and becomes strangulated, the patient may experience chest pain, syncope, or sudden death. Surgery may be required in cases of cardiac herniation to close or enlarge the pericardial defect.

Types and Associations

The most common type is congenital absence of the left pericardium with preservation of the right pericardium (as in the case shown). Occasionally, congenital absence of the pericardium is associated with other congenital heart defects, including atrial septal defect, patent ductus arteriosus, mitral valve stenosis, and tetralogy of Fallot.

Imaging Findings and Diagnosis

Chest radiographs typically demonstrate the characteristic leftward deviation and rotation of the heart without deviation of the remainder of the mediastinum and prominence of the left atrial appendage (Fig. A). These features are also seen on CT and MRI (Figs. B and C). Demonstration of lung interposed between the aorta and pulmonary artery on CT or MRI confirms the diagnosis (Fig. D).

Notes

Challenge

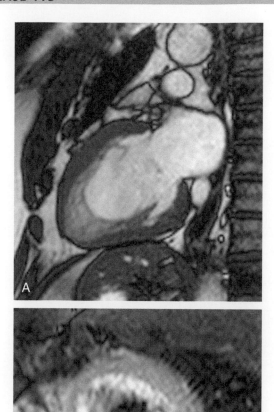

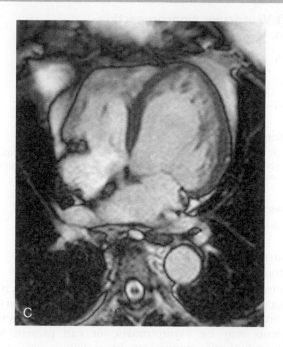

History: No patient history is available.

1. What should be included in the differential diagnosis of high signal within the outer aspect of the left ventricular cavity on black blood MRI? (Choose all that apply.)
   A. Myocarditis
   B. Left ventricular noncompaction
   C. Sarcoidosis
   D. Myocardial contusion

2. What is responsible for the hyperintense signal at the periphery of the left ventricular cavity on the short-axis black blood image (Fig. B)?
   A. Slow or stagnant flow
   B. Myocardial edema
   C. Fast-moving blood
   D. Myocardial contusion

3. Which of the following is the most likely clinical presentation for this patient?
   A. A 16-year-old boy presents with chest pain and fever following an upper respiratory tract infection.
   B. A 40-year-old man presents with acute pleuritic chest pain and diffuse ST segment elevation on all ECG leads.
   C. A 40-year-old man presents with cardiac arrhythmia and history of a cardiac thromboembolic event.
   D. A 30-year-old woman presents with cough, and a chest radiograph obtained at the time of admission shows right paratracheal and symmetric bilateral hilar lymphadenopathy.

4. What is the MRI criterion for diagnosing this condition?
   A. An elevated noncompacted/compacted myocardial layer (NC/C) ratio measured at end-systole
   B. An elevated NC/C ratio measured at end-diastole
   C. A reduced NC/C ratio measured at end-systole
   D. A reduced NC/C ratio measured at end-diastole

CASE 118

Left Ventricular Noncompaction

1. A, B, C, and D

2. A

3. C

4. B

Reference

Yun H, Zeng MS, Jin H, et al: Isolated noncompaction of ventricular myocardium: a magnetic resonance imaging study of 11 patients, *Korean J Radiol* 12(6):686-692, 2011.

Cross-Reference

Cardiac Imaging: The REQUISITES, ed 3, p 54.

Comment

Pathophysiology

Ventricular noncompaction is a more recently described primary cardiomyopathy thought to be secondary to an arrest in myocardial development and compaction. Patients may be asymptomatic or can present with tachyarrhythmia, congestive heart failure, or cardiac thromboembolism. Ventricular noncompaction may be seen with other cardiac abnormalities including atrial septal defect, ventricular septal defect, partial anomalous pulmonary venous return, pulmonic stenosis, and Ebstein anomaly.

Imaging Findings, Diagnostic Criteria, and Therapy

Ventricular noncompaction most commonly affects the left ventricle. Cardiac MRI and CT findings include prominent trabeculations, deep intertrabecular recesses that communicate with the ventricular cavity, and an elevated NC/C ratio (Figs. A-C). There may be adjacent wall motion abnormality and transmural or subendocardial late gadolinium enhancement. The MRI criterion for diagnosing pathologic left ventricular noncompaction is an elevated NC/C ratio greater than 2.3 measured in end-diastole. Treatment involves aspirin in all patients to reduce the risk of systemic embolism and beta blockers and angiotensin-converting enzyme (ACE) inhibitors in patients with heart dysfunction.

Notes

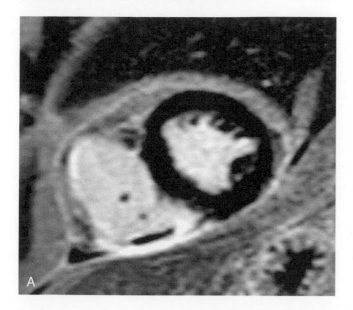

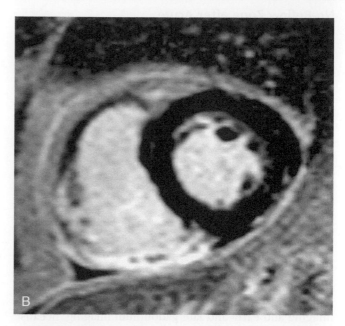

History: A patient undergoes cardiac MRI 5 days after percutaneous intervention for ST segment elevation myocardial infarction.

1. What should be included in the differential diagnosis for myocardial late gadolinium enhancement? (Choose all that apply.)
   A. Myocardial infarction
   B. Myocardial sarcoidosis
   C. Myocardial amyloidosis
   D. Hypertrophic cardiomyopathy
   E. Dilated cardiomyopathy

2. What MRI sequence is shown in Figs. A and B?
   A. Black blood MRI
   B. Phase contrast MRI
   C. Steady-state free precession (SSFP) MRI
   D. Inversion recovery late gadolinium enhancement MRI

3. What is the most likely cause of the hyperintense signal within the right ventricular wall?
   A. Myocardial infarction
   B. Myocardial contusion
   C. Amyloidosis
   D. Hypertrophic cardiomyopathy

4. Which cardiac MRI sequence can identify microvascular obstruction?
   A. Cine steady-state free precession
   B. Velocity-encoded cine phase contrast MRI
   C. First-pass perfusion imaging
   D. Black blood imaging

No-Reflow Zone after Acute Myocardial Infarction

1. A, B, C, D, and E

2. D

3. A

4. C

References

Ito H: No-reflow phenomenon and prognosis in patients with acute myocardial infarction, *Nat Clin Pract Cardiovasc Med* 3(9):499–506, 2006.

Mather AN, Lockie T, Nagel E, et al: Appearance of microvascular obstruction on high resolution first-pass perfusion, early and late gadolinium enhancement CMR in patients with acute myocardial infarction, *J Cardiovasc Magn Reson* 11:33, 2009.

Comment

Imaging

No-reflow zone can be detected on first-pass perfusion imaging and early and late gadolinium imaging. Because contrast material cannot reach the myocardium owing to microvascular obstruction, it remains dark on all post-gadolinium sequences (Figs. A and B). First-pass perfusion imaging is the most accurate predictor of the size of a no-reflow zone. Late gadolinium images likely underestimate the degree of microvascular obstruction because contrast material often diffuses into the edge of the no-reflow zone.

Pathophysiology and Prognosis

Cardiac MRI is a useful prognostic tool after intervention for acute ST segment elevation myocardial infarction because it directly quantifies the volume of infarcted myocardium and the extent of microvascular obstruction. After myocardial infarction, no-reflow zone is caused by a breakdown or obstruction of the coronary microvasculature in the territory supplied by the previously obstructed coronary artery. The presence of a no-reflow zone is a poor prognostic indicator; patients have an increased future risk of lower ejection fraction, more ventricular remodeling, and higher risk of death.

Notes

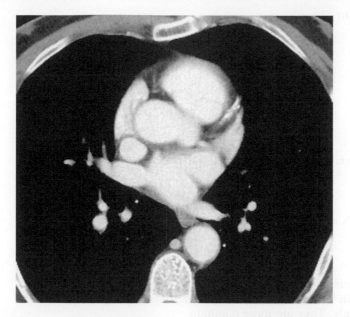

History: A 60-year-old man with a malignant peripheral nerve sheath tumor involving the lumbar spine undergoes surveillance CT.

1. What should be included in the differential diagnosis for a saccular outpouching from a vessel? (Choose all that apply.)
   A. Mycotic aneurysm
   B. Annuloaortic ectasia
   C. Traumatic pseudoaneurysm
   D. Atherosclerotic aneurysm

2. What is the most likely diagnosis?
   A. Sinus of Valsalva aneurysm
   B. Atherosclerotic aneurysm
   C. Traumatic pseudoaneurysm
   D. Annuloaortic ectasia

3. Where is the most common site of rupture of this entity?
   A. Pericardium
   B. Right-sided chamber
   C. Left-sided chamber
   D. Pleural cavity

4. What is the most common complication from rupture?
   A. Hemothorax
   B. Aortic dissection
   C. Cardiac tamponade
   D. Congestive heart failure

CASE 120

Sinus of Valsalva Aneurysm

1. A, C, and D

2. A

3. B

4. D

Reference

Bricker AO, Avutu B, Mohammed TL, et al: Valsalva sinus aneurysms: findings at CT and MR imaging, *Radiographics* 30(1):99-110, 2010.

Cross-Reference

Cardiac Imaging: The REQUISITES, ed 3, pp 389-392.

Comment

Epidemiology

Sinus of Valsalva aneurysms are rare congenital or acquired lesions that occur in 0.09% of patients as determined in a large autopsy study. They are more common in men and people of Asian descent. The right coronary cusp is affected in most cases (72%) followed by the noncoronary cusp (22%). When symptoms exist, they are often secondary to rupture or mass effect on a coronary artery, superior vena cava, or ventricular outflow tract. Sinus of Valsalva aneurysms most commonly rupture into the right ventricle followed by the right atrium. Rupture into a cardiac chamber causes an aortocardiac shunt with the eventual development of congestive heart failure. Large nonruptured aneurysms may cause mass effect on adjacent structures or lead to aortic regurgitation.

Diagnosis and Treatment

Sinus of Valsalva aneurysms are most commonly diagnosed with echocardiography. Occasionally, CT or MRI may be used in difficult cases, or aneurysms may be discovered on imaging performed for other reasons. The imaging criteria to diagnose this condition include a saccular shape, aneurysm origin above the aortic anulus, and a normal dimension of the aortic root and ascending aorta. Definitive treatment is cardiopulmonary bypass surgery or percutaneous repair.

Imaging

Contrast-enhanced CT through the level of the aortic root shows a saccular outpouching arising from the left sinus of Valsalva (Figure). The adjacent aortic root and ascending aorta have a normal diameter. No communication with the ventricle is present. These findings are consistent with an unruptured left coronary sinus of Valsalva aneurysm.

Notes

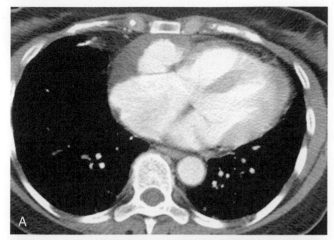

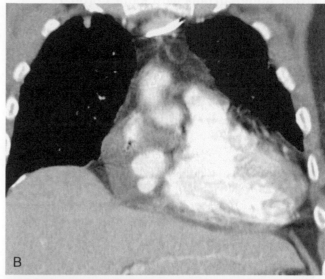

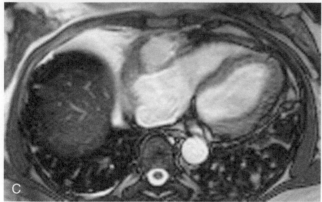

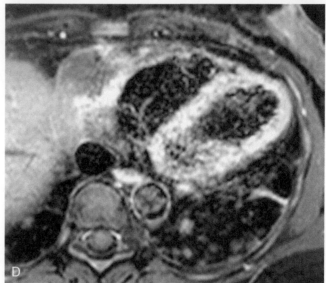

History: A 65-year-old woman presents with chest heaviness and abnormality on initial chest radiograph.

1. What should be included in the differential diagnosis for a cardiac mass? (Choose all that apply.)
   A. Thrombus
   B. Angiosarcoma
   C. Myxoma
   D. Melanoma metastasis

2. What is the most common cardiac mass?
   A. Thrombus
   B. Benign primary cardiac tumor
   C. Malignant primary cardiac tumor
   D. Metastasis

3. Which imaging finding is more suggestive of a benign cardiac tumor?
   A. Infiltrative appearance
   B. Lung nodules
   C. Involvement of one cardiac chamber
   D. Extension outside the heart

4. What is the most likely diagnosis given the absence of a known primary?
   A. Liposarcoma
   B. Thrombus
   C. Myxoma
   D. Angiosarcoma

CASE 121

Cardiac Angiosarcoma with Right Coronary Artery Pseudoaneurysm

1. A, B, C, and D

2. A

3. C

4. D

References

Berry MF, Williams M, Welsby I, et al: Cardiac angiosarcoma presenting with right coronary artery pseudoaneurysm, *J Cardiothorac Vasc Anesth* 24(4):633–635, 2010.

Randhawa K, Ganeshan A, Hoey ET: Magnetic resonance imaging of cardiac tumors: part 2, malignant tumors and tumor-like conditions, *Curr Probl Diagn Radiol* 40(4):169–179, 2011.

Cross-Reference

Cardiac Imaging: The REQUISITES, ed 3, pp 281–282.

Comment

Epidemiology and Prognosis

Most cardiac tumors (98%) are metastases from extracardiac primaries. Angiosarcoma is the most common primary malignant cardiac tumor. It is usually an infiltrative right atrial free wall mass. It often extends outside the heart and may involve more than one cardiac chamber. Rarely, it can lead to a right coronary artery pseudoaneurysm as shown in this case. Prognosis is poor with median survival less than 1 year in patients with metastatic disease.

Imaging

Cardiac CT images (Figs. A and B) show an infiltrative mass involving the free wall of the right atrium and right ventricle. Within the mass is a round collection of contrast material, which is separate from the cardiac chambers located in the right atrioventricular groove. An axial bright blood image shows right atrial free wall thickening and a right coronary artery pseudoaneurysm (Fig. C). A black blood image obtained after gadolinium administration (Fig. D) shows enhancement of the right atrial free wall mass. This patient had multiple pulmonary nodules, and biopsy of these yielded a diagnosis of angiosarcoma.

Notes

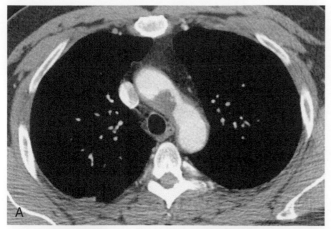

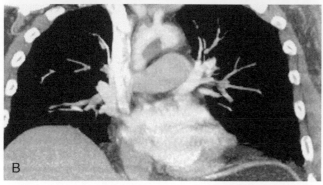

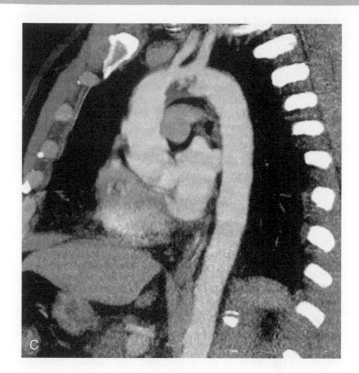

History: A 35-year-old man presents with peripheral limb ischemia and stroke.

1. What should be included in the differential diagnosis? (Choose all that apply.)
   A. Thromboembolism
   B. Vasculitis
   C. Tumor
   D. Atherosclerotic plaque

2. Which of the following conditions is likely associated with this lesion?
   A. Stroke
   B. Benign clinical course
   C. Pulmonary embolism
   D. Limbic encephalitis

3. Which of the following would be the most likely diagnosis if this patient also had bilateral heterogeneously enhancing adrenal masses?
   A. Vasculitis
   B. Tumor
   C. Atheromatous plaque
   D. Thromboembolism

4. Aortic intimal sarcoma most commonly occurs in what gender and age group?
   A. Elderly men
   B. Elderly women
   C. No gender predilection
   D. Children

CASE 122

Aortic Intimal Sarcoma

1. C and D

2. A

3. B

4. A

References

Crone KG, Bhalla S, Pfeifer JD: Aortic intimal sarcoma detected on helical CT, *J Thorac Imaging* 19(2):120-122, 2004.

Kato W, Usui A, Oshima H, et al: Primary aortic intimal sarcoma, *Gen Thorac Cardiovasc Surg* 56(5):236-238, 2008.

Comment

Epidemiology and Treatment

Aortic intimal sarcoma is an exceptionally rare tumor of vascular origin. Most reported cases originate in the abdominal aorta. This tumor is often diagnosed late because both clinical presentation and imaging findings mimic atheromatous plaque. Symptoms are usually secondary to thromboembolic events with tumor embolism causing claudication, bowel ischemia, renal infarcts, or stroke. Prognosis is poor because the tumor tends to metastasize early. Treatment is surgical resection in patients without evidence of metastatic disease.

Imaging

This entity should be considered when an irregularly shaped lesion arises from the aortic wall. There is no evidence of dissection or penetrating ulcer. The most helpful imaging finding is the presence of an associated paraaortic mass that is contiguous with the intraluminal lesion. As in this case, the diagnosis is usually made at the time of surgery because the lesion is thought to represent an atheromatous plaque.

Coronal, axial, and oblique sagittal images (Figs. A-C) show an irregularly shaped mass arising from the inferior wall of the proximal aortic arch. The patient in this case presented with a frontal lobe infarct and a cold, ischemic left arm from tumor embolism into the left brachial artery. The preoperative diagnosis was a large atheroma in the aortic arch. Pathology showed the lesion was an intimal sarcoma.

Notes

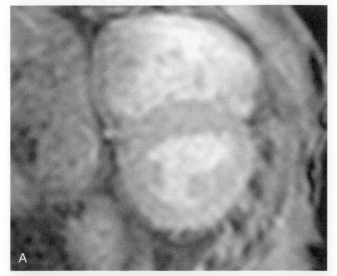

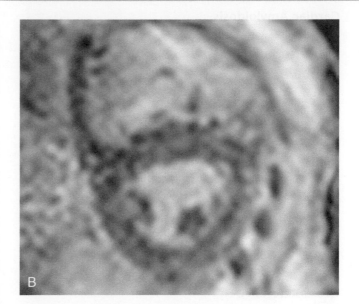

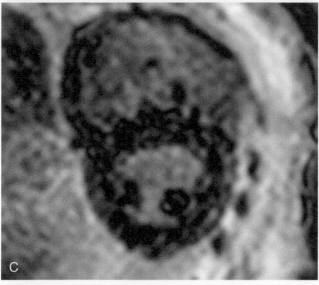

History: A 50-year-old man presents with lower extremity edema and progressive dyspnea on exertion.

1. What should be included in the differential diagnosis for restrictive cardiomyopathy? (Choose all that apply.)
   A. Tuberculosis infection
   B. Radiation therapy
   C. Amyloidosis
   D. Doxorubicin (Adriamycin) therapy
   E. Sarcoidosis

2. What imaging sequence is shown in Figs. A-C?
   A. Steady-state free precession (SSFP)
   B. Look locker (cine inversion recovery)
   C. Black blood
   D. Phase contrast

3. What is abnormal about the images?
   A. Nothing
   B. Myocardium is nulled before blood pool.
   C. Intramyocardial mass
   D. Transmural late gadolinium enhancement in Fig. A

4. What additional finding on late gadolinium enhancement MRI would support the most likely diagnosis based on these figures?
   A. Patchy enhancement not corresponding to an arterial distribution
   B. Transmural enhancement in the territory of the left anterior descending (LAD) coronary artery
   C. No late gadolinium enhancement
   D. Diffuse subendocardial enhancement

Cardiac Amyloidosis

1. B, C, and E

2. B

3. B

4. D

References

Maceira AM, Joshi J, Prasad SK, et al: Cardiovascular magnetic resonance in cardiac amyloidosis, *Circulation* 111(2):186-193, 2005.

Ordovas KG, Higgins CB: Delayed contrast enhancement on MR images of myocardium: past, present, future, *Radiology* 261(2):358-374, 2011.

Vogelsberg H, Mahrholdt H, Deluigi CC, et al: Cardiovascular magnetic resonance in clinically suspected cardiac amyloidosis: noninvasive imaging compared to endomyocardial biopsy, *J Am Coll Cardiol* 51(10):1022-1030, 2008.

Cross-Reference

Cardiac Imaging: The REQUISITES, ed 3, p 286 (figure only).

Comment

Overview

Cardiac amyloidosis is a common cause of secondary restrictive cardiomyopathy. Amyloid fibrillar proteins deposit in myocardium and lead to reduced ventricular compliance and diastolic function. Patients present with restrictive or constrictive physiology. Common symptoms include lower extremity edema, ascites, and dyspnea. MRI can differentiate constrictive pericarditis from restrictive cardiomyopathy. Constrictive pericarditis typically has pericardial thickening greater than or equal to 4 mm, whereas restrictive cardiomyopathy does not. Many causes of restrictive cardiomyopathy, such as amyloidosis, have characteristic appearances on late gadolinium enhancement imaging.

Evaluation

Abnormal myocardial nulling before blood pool nulling is likely secondary to cardiac deposition of amyloid protein. Amyloid deposition disrupts gadolinium kinetics and is responsible for loss of contrast between normal and abnormal myocardium when patients undergo late gadolinium enhancement imaging 8 minutes or longer after contrast agent injection. In patients with suspected cardiac amyloidosis, late gadolinium enhancement imaging ideally should be performed 5 to 8 minutes after contrast agent administration to maximize the difference between normal and abnormal myocardium. Diffuse subendocardial enhancement affecting the right and left ventricles is a characteristic enhancement pattern seen in cardiac amyloidosis. An additional finding includes wall thickening in affected myocardium.

Imaging

Three images from a short-axis inversion recovery look locker sequence (Figs. A-C) show diffuse nulling (black signal) of the myocardium before blood pool nulling. Normal myocardium is typically nulled (black signal) after the blood pool (opposite of the present case).

Notes

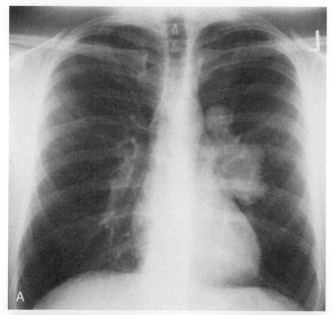

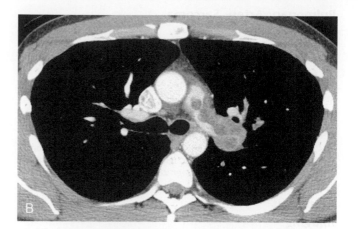

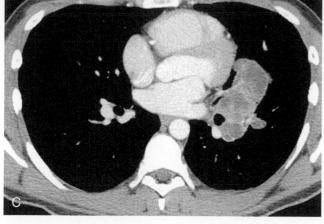

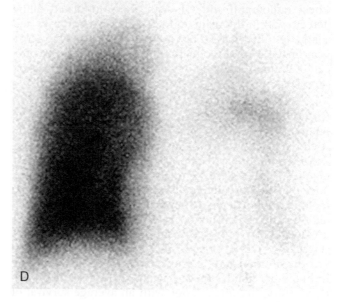

History: A patient presents with chest pain.

1. What are potential causes for the perfusion abnormality in Fig. D? (Choose all that apply.)
   A. Pulmonary embolism
   B. Tumor
   C. Fibrosing mediastinitis
   D. Emphysema
   E. Pneumonectomy

2. What is the most likely diagnosis?
   A. Pulmonary embolism
   B. Pneumonectomy
   C. Tumor
   D. Sarcoidosis

3. Which symptom or CT feature favors a pulmonary artery sarcoma over a pulmonary embolism?
   A. Bilaterality
   B. Expansion of the pulmonary artery
   C. Dyspnea and cough
   D. Unilateral lung hypoperfusion on ventilation/ perfusion scan

4. What is the most common cause of a unilateral hilar mass?
   A. Lung cancer
   B. Sarcoidosis
   C. Castleman disease
   D. Bronchogenic cyst

CASE 124

Pulmonary Artery Sarcoma

1. A, B, C, and E

2. C

3. B

4. A

Reference

Yi CA, Lee KS, Choe YH, et al: Computed tomography in pulmonary artery sarcoma: distinguishing features from pulmonary embolic disease, *J Comput Assist Tomogr* 28(1):34–39, 2004.

Comment

Imaging

Chest radiograph and CT scan show lobulated filling defects within the main and left pulmonary arteries and a large left hilar mass (Figs. A-C). A corresponding perfusion image from a technetium-99m-labeled macroaggregated albumin study shows minimal left lung perfusion (Fig. D).

Differential Diagnosis

Pulmonary artery sarcoma is extremely rare, and prospective diagnosis is difficult. The main differential diagnosis is pulmonary embolism. Both conditions may manifest with dyspnea, cough, and chest pain. CT findings that are predictive of pulmonary artery sarcoma include a filling defect occupying the entire lumen of the main or proximal pulmonary arteries, expansion of the involved artery, or extraluminal extension of tumor (Figs. A-C). Other clues to the diagnosis include unilateral distribution and heterogeneous enhancement of the intraluminal filling defect (Fig. B). Prognosis of pulmonary artery sarcoma is poor with an average survival of 12 months after symptom onset.

Notes

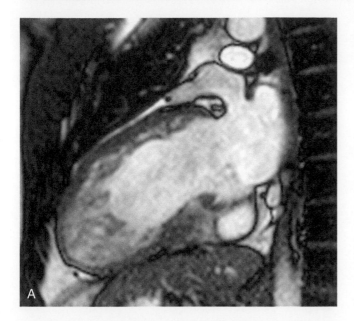

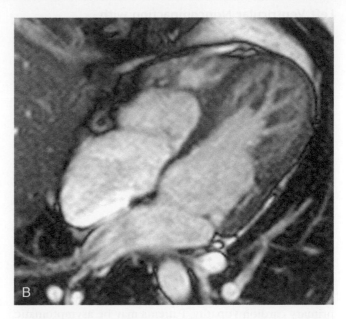

History: No patient history is available.

1. Which of the following valves can be evaluated on the MRI four-chamber view? (Choose all that apply.)
   A. Mitral
   B. Tricuspid
   C. Aortic
   D. Pulmonic

2. What imaging planes are shown?
   A. Vertical long-axis and four-chamber
   B. Vertical long-axis and left ventricular outflow tract
   C. Left ventricular outflow tract and four-chamber
   D. Right ventricular outflow tract and short-axis

3. Which valve is abnormal?
   A. Mitral
   B. Tricuspid
   C. Pulmonic
   D. Aortic

4. In addition to the abnormal valve, what is the other finding?
   A. Noncompaction
   B. Cardiac mass
   C. Myocardial infarction
   D. Pericardial effusion

Left Ventricular Noncompaction with Ebstein Anomaly

1. A and B

2. A

3. B

4. A

Reference

Betrián Blasco P, Gallardo Agromayor E: Ebstein's anomaly and left ventricular noncompaction association, *Int J Cardiol* 119(2):264–265, 2007.

Cross-Reference

Cardiac Imaging: The REQUISITES, ed 3, p 54.

Comment

Presentation and Associations

Ventricular noncompaction is a more recently described primary cardiomyopathy. Patients may be asymptomatic or may present with tachyarrhythmia, congestive heart failure, or cardiac thromboembolism. Pathologic noncompaction is occasionally associated with other cardiac conditions, including atrial septal defect, ventricular septal defect, pulmonic stenosis, partial anomalous pulmonary venous return, and Ebstein anomaly.

Imaging

Cine steady-state free precession (SSFP) vertical long-axis and four-chamber images show prominent trabeculation with a distinct two-layered appearance of the left and right ventricular myocardium (Figs. A and B). There are deep intertrabecular recesses, and the measured ratio of noncompacted to compacted myocardium is elevated, measuring greater than 2.3 at end-diastole. This appearance fulfills the MRI diagnostic criterion for pathologic ventricular noncompaction. An additional observation is ventricular displacement of the tricuspid valve with respect to the mitral valve, consistent with Ebstein anomaly (Fig. B).

Notes

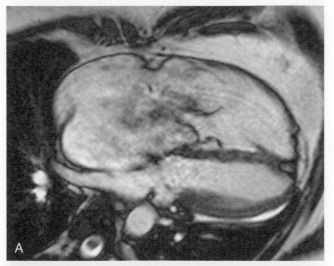

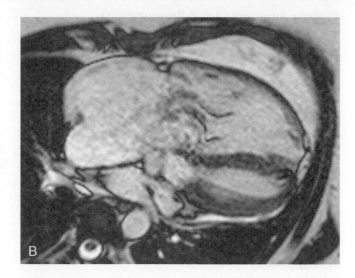

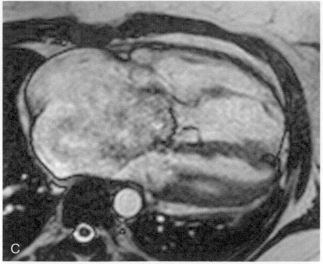

History: A 39-year-old woman presents with increasing exercise intolerance, palpitations, fatigue, and valve abnormality seen on a recent transthoracic echocardiogram.

1. What are causes of right heart failure? (Choose all that apply.)
   A. Left heart failure
   B. Emphysema
   C. Idiopathic pulmonary fibrosis
   D. Chronic pulmonary embolism
   E. Congenital pulmonary stenosis

2. What is the main finding involving the cardiac chambers?
   A. Dilation of the right-sided chambers
   B. Dilation of left-sided chambers
   C. Four-chamber dilation
   D. Multiple cardiac masses

3. What valve abnormality would explain the dilated chambers?
   A. Mitral regurgitation
   B. Aortic regurgitation
   C. Tricuspid regurgitation
   D. Pulmonic regurgitation

4. What is the most likely diagnosis?
   A. Pulmonary hypertension
   B. Rheumatic heart disease
   C. Left ventricular failure
   D. Ebstein anomaly

CASE 126

Ebstein Anomaly (Adult Presentation)

1. A, B, C, D, and E

2. A

3. C

4. D

Reference

Yalonetsky S, Tobler D, Greutmann M, et al: Cardiac magnetic resonance imaging and the assessment of Ebstein anomaly in adults, *Am J Cardiol* 107(5):767–773, 2011.

Cross-Reference

Cardiac Imaging: The REQUISITES, ed 3, pp 206–207.

Comment

Description

Ebstein anomaly is a rare congenital heart disease that usually results in cyanosis early in life. This anomaly is characterized by varying degrees of ventricular displacement of the tricuspid valve leaflets, resulting in a common ventriculoatrial chamber and often severe tricuspid regurgitation. The tricuspid anulus is not displaced. Over time, there is progressive dilation of the right-sided chambers, which leads to increased tricuspid regurgitation and further chamber dilation. Occasionally, the degree of ventricular displacement of the tricuspid leaflets is mild, resulting in less tricuspid regurgitation and less right atrial dilation. These patients commonly present later in life and sometimes as adults.

Imaging

Cine steady-state free precession (SSFP) images (Figs. A-C) in the four-chamber view show dilation of the right atrium and right ventricle. The tricuspid valve leaflets are displaced toward the right ventricle, and there is associated severe tricuspid regurgitation, with the tricuspid regurgitant fraction measuring 74%. This patient had a late presentation of Ebstein anomaly. She noted fatigue beginning in her early 20s, which progressed to exercise intolerance and lower extremity edema.

Role of MRI in Adults

Echocardiography allows precise morphologic and functional evaluation of the right ventricle in children with Ebstein anomaly. This evaluation is important because right ventricular size is directly correlated to patient outcomes and prognosis. In adults, the acoustic windows needed to image the right atrium and ventricle on echocardiography may be inadequate or allow incomplete visualization of the chambers. MRI provides the same information as echocardiography and gives more reliable and reproducible information in patients with limited acoustic windows. MRI can assess right ventricular size and function and accurately quantitate the volume of tricuspid regurgitation, which has a direct impact on the timing of valvular surgery in these patients.

Notes

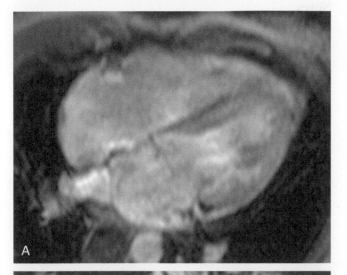

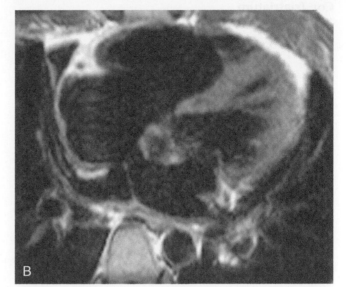

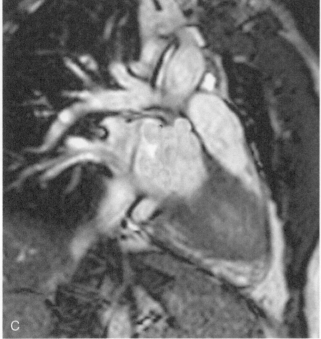

History: A 34-year-old man is referred for MRI after an echocardiogram shows a patent foramen ovale and a thin membrane within the left atrium.

1. What are causes of pulmonary edema? (Choose all that apply.)
   A. Right heart failure
   B. Left heart failure
   C. Mitral stenosis
   D. Large volume thoracentesis

2. What is the finding in the left atrium?
   A. Thin membrane
   B. Pedunculated mass arising from the septum
   C. Fat infiltration of the septum
   D. Infiltrative mass

3. What is the diagnosis?
   A. Cor triatriatum
   B. Myxoma
   C. Lipomatous hypertrophy
   D. Angiosarcoma

4. How is this condition managed when it is discovered in the neonatal period?
   A. "Don't touch" lesion
   B. Afterload-reducing medications
   C. Follow-up imaging
   D. Surgical resection

CASE 127

Cor Triatriatum
1. B, C, and D

2. A

3. A

4. D

References
Holloway BJ, Agarwal PP: Incidental cor triatriatum discovered on multidetector computed tomography, *J Thorac Imaging* 26(2):W45–W47, 2011.

Krasemann Z, Scheld HH, Tjan TD, et al: Cor triatriatum: short review of the literature upon ten new cases, *Herz* 32(6):506–510, 2007.

Su CS, Tsai IC, Lin WW, et al: Usefulness of multidetector-row computed tomography in evaluating adult cor triatriatum, *Tex Heart Inst J* 35(3):349–351, 2008.

Cross-Reference
Cardiac Imaging: The REQUISITES, ed 3, pp 190–191.

Comment
Imaging
Cine steady-state free precession (SSFP) and black blood four-chamber images show a thin membrane in the posterior left atrium extending to the interatrial septum. The membrane divides the atrium into two chambers separating the right from the left pulmonary venous inflow (Figs. A and B).

Description
Cor triatriatum, also known as the triatrial heart, is a congenital heart defect characterized by a thin membrane dividing either the right or the left atrium. In most patients, either single or multiple fenestrations within the membrane allow unimpeded blood flow. In adults, the fenestration is often large, and the heart defect is of little or no clinical significance and rarely causes symptoms. When the defect causes symptoms, it mimics the clinical presentation of mitral stenosis. In infants and children, the fenestration is often small or absent, leading to dyspnea, failure to thrive, and cyanosis.

Diagnosis
Cor triatriatum is most commonly diagnosed with echocardiography; transesophageal echocardiography is more sensitive than transthoracic echocardiography. This entity is increasingly being diagnosed with the aid of CT or MRI. These modalities also aid in diagnosis of other associated congenital heart defects. Cine SSFP MRI is helpful in assessing for turbulent flow through the fenestration as a marker of flow disturbance.

Significance in Adults
Cor triatriatum is an incidental finding of no consequence if the fenestration is large and discovered in adults. Cor triatriatum in infants and children is surgically corrected when the fenestration is small or absent. Patient prognosis is excellent if there are no coexisting heart defects.

Notes

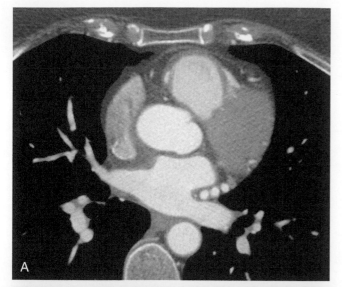

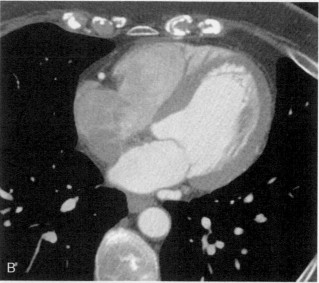

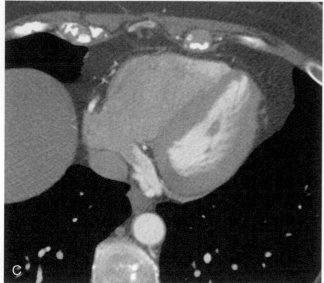

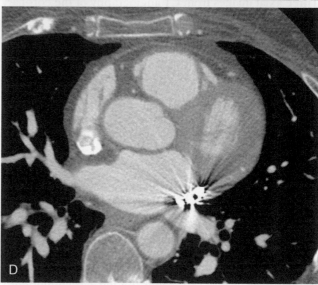

History: A 54-year-old woman presents with dyspnea, chest pain, and exertional syncope. The symptoms have been ongoing for 15 years and occur only with exertion.

1. What should be included in the differential diagnosis for a dilated coronary artery? (Choose all that apply.)
   A. Atherosclerosis
   B. Anomalous left coronary artery from the pulmonary artery
   C. Fistula
   D. Takayasu arteritis

2. Which coronary artery is enlarged?
   A. Right
   B. Left main
   C. Left anterior descending
   D. Left circumflex

3. Which structure is opacified at the same time as the left circumflex coronary artery at the inferior aspect of the heart (Fig. C)?
   A. Coronary sinus
   B. Great cardiac vein
   C. Middle cardiac vein
   D. Small cardiac vein

4. What is the abnormality affecting the left circumflex coronary artery?
   A. Dissection
   B. Aneurysm
   C. Fistula
   D. Anomalous course

CASE 128

Left Circumflex Coronary Artery Fistula to Coronary Sinus

1. A, B, C, and D

2. D

3. A

4. C

Reference

Díaz-Zamudio M, Bacilio-Pérez U, Herrera-Zarza MC, et al: Coronary artery aneurysms and ectasia: role of coronary CT angiography, *Radiographics* 29(7):1939-1954, 2009.

Cross-Reference

Cardiac Imaging: The REQUISITES, ed 3, pp 228-229, 253.

Comment

Imaging

Three axial images from CT angiography of the coronary arteries show marked dilation and tortuosity of the circumflex coronary artery (Figs. A-C). There is contrast opacification of the distal coronary sinus (Fig. C) without opacification of the more proximal great cardiac vein; this is consistent with a coronary artery fistula to the coronary sinus. Syncope in this patient was thought to be secondary to a coronary steal phenomenon that occurred with exercise, and she was treated successfully with coil embolization of the distal circumflex coronary artery (Fig. D).

Description

A coronary fistula is usually a congenital connection between a coronary artery and cardiac chamber or great vessel that bypasses the myocardial capillaries. Coronary fistulas can rarely occur after myocardial biopsy or open heart surgery. The right coronary artery is affected in most cases (52%), followed by the left anterior descending coronary artery (30%) and the left circumflex coronary artery (18%). In most patients (90%), the fistula drains into the right circulation causing a left-to-right shunt.

Notes

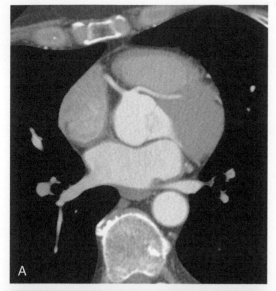

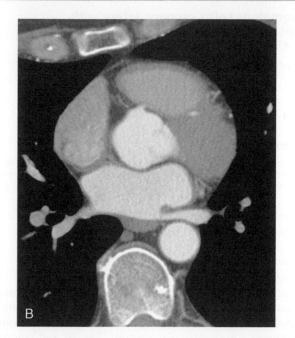

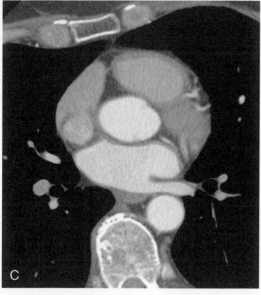

History: A 54-year-old quadriplegic man presents with severe chest heaviness.

1. What are causes of sudden cardiac death in adolescents and young adults? (Choose all that apply.)
   A. Hypertrophic cardiomyopathy
   B. Anomalous left coronary artery
   C. Long QT syndrome
   D. Athlete's heart

2. What is the anomaly?
   A. Anomalous left coronary artery from the pulmonary artery
   B. Anomalous right coronary artery from the left sinus of Valsalva
   C. Anomalous left coronary artery from the right sinus of Valsalva
   D. Benign anomalous variant

3. What course does the anomalous vessel take?
   A. Prepulmonic
   B. Retroaortic
   C. Septal
   D. Interarterial

4. What is the usual treatment or next imaging step for an anomalous left coronary artery with a septal course?
   A. "Don't touch" lesion
   B. Stress testing
   C. Stenting
   D. Surgery

Anomalous Left Coronary Artery with Septal Course

Notes

1. A, B, and C

2. C

3. C

4. B

Reference

Young PM, Gerber TC, Williamson EE, et al: Cardiac imaging: part 2, normal, variant, and anomalous configurations of the coronary vasculature, *AJR Am J Roentgenol* 197(4):816–826, 2011.

Cross-Reference

Cardiac Imaging: The REQUISITES, ed 3, pp 225–228.

Comment

Imaging

CT angiography of the coronary arteries shows an anomalous left coronary artery arising from the right sinus of Valsalva (Figs. A-C). The artery courses superiorly through the upper interventricular septum (Fig. B) and emerges to trifurcate into the circumflex, ramus intermedius, and left anterior descending coronary arteries. This patient was unable to undergo stress testing or surgery because of clinical deterioration unrelated to the anomalous coronary artery.

Overview

An ectopic coronary origin is an important anomaly to recognize given the increased risk of sudden cardiac death in certain variants. There are four paths that the anomalous vessel can take to supply its myocardial territory:

1. Retroaortic: This variant is benign and is not associated with an increased risk of sudden cardiac death.

2. Prepulmonic: This is also a benign variant. This vessel has an increased risk of accelerated atherosclerosis and can be injured if the patient undergoes median sternotomy, especially for repair of tetralogy of Fallot.

3. Interarterial: This is the so-called malignant variant in which the artery courses between the aorta and pulmonary artery. Patients are at an increased risk of sudden cardiac death and are usually treated surgically with bypass grafting or reimplantation of the anomalous artery.

4. Septal: This variant is often confused with the interarterial course; however, in the septal path, the artery travels through the myocardium in the proximal interventricular septum. Stress testing helps determine the clinical significance of this lesion. Patients who develop ischemia are treated surgically.

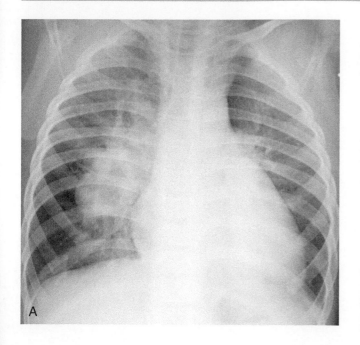

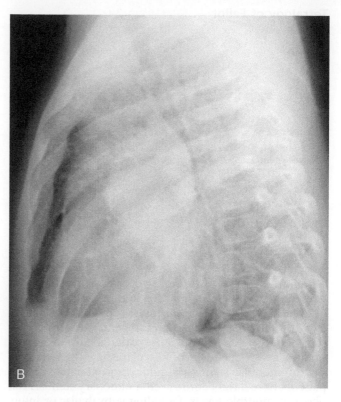

History: A child presents with shortness of breath.

1. What should be included in the differential diagnosis? (Choose all that apply.)
   A. Pulmonary hypertension
   B. Pulmonary artery aneurysms
   C. Tetralogy of Fallot with absent pulmonary valve
   D. Pulmonary stenosis

2. Which vessel or vessels are enlarged?
   A. Aorta
   B. Pulmonary arteries
   C. Pulmonary veins
   D. Superior vena cava

3. This patient has tetralogy of Fallot. What is the most likely diagnosis?
   A. Right aortic arch
   B. "Pink tet"
   C. Coronary artery anomaly
   D. Absent pulmonary valve

4. What is the cause of large lung volumes in these patients?
   A. Emphysema
   B. Bronchiectasis
   C. Infections
   D. Airway compression

CASE 130

Tetralogy of Fallot

1. A, B, and C

2. B

3. D

4. D

Reference

Kirshbom PM, Kogon BE: Tetralogy of Fallot with absent pulmonary valve syndrome, *Semin Thorac Cardiovasc Surg Pediatr Card Surg Annu* 7:65-71, 2004.

Cross-Reference

Cardiac Imaging: The REQUISITES, ed 3, pp 359-367.

Comment

Overview

Tetralogy of Fallot is the most common cyanotic congenital heart disease in children and adults. The lesions of tetralogy of Fallot are ventricular septal defect, pulmonary infundibular stenosis, right ventricular hypertrophy, and overriding aorta. Most patients have decreased pulmonary vascularity, but vascularity can be normal if the infundibular stenosis is mild. Approximately 25% of patients have a right aortic arch. Pulmonary stenosis can occur at multiple levels, including subvalvular or infundibular (most common), valvular, supravalvular, and in peripheral pulmonary arteries. The chest radiograph typically demonstrates decreased vascularity, concavity of the pulmonary artery segment, and sometimes an upturned cardiac apex.

Clinical Features

Tetralogy of Fallot with absent pulmonary valve syndrome is characterized by a hypoplastic pulmonary annulus containing primitive valve tissue and aneurysmal dilation of the pulmonary arteries. The other lesions of tetralogy also exist in these patients. The marked pulmonary artery enlargement causes large airway compression, leading to early onset of respiratory distress.

Imaging

Unlike other types of tetralogy of Fallot, chest radiographs typically demonstrate marked dilation of the main, left, and right pulmonary arteries (Figs. A and B). The lung volumes frequently are large, a consequence of tracheobronchial compression.

Notes

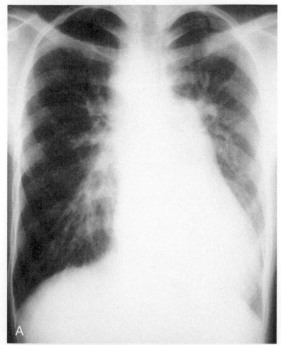

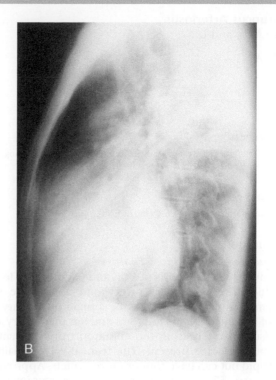

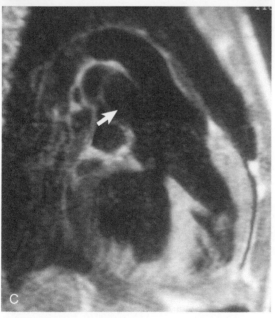

History: A patient presents with cyanosis.

1. What should be included in the differential diagnosis in a patient with cyanosis and increased pulmonary vascularity? (Choose all that apply.)
   A. Transposition of the great arteries
   B. Total anomalous pulmonary venous connection
   C. Tetralogy of Fallot
   D. Truncus arteriosus

2. What structure is indicated by the arrow in Fig. C?
   A. Pulmonary artery
   B. Ascending aorta
   C. Aortic arch
   D. Superior vena cava

3. What is the most likely diagnosis?
   A. Transposition of the great arteries
   B. Total anomalous pulmonary venous connection
   C. Tetralogy of Fallot
   D. Truncus arteriosus

4. What other cyanotic heart disease is most strongly associated with a right aortic arch?
   A. Transposition of the great arteries
   B. Total anomalous pulmonary venous connection
   C. Tetralogy of Fallot
   D. Ebstein anomaly

Truncus Arteriosus

1. A, B, and D

2. A

3. D

4. C

Reference

Johnson TR: Conotruncal cardiac defects: a clinical imaging perspective, *Pediatr Cardiol* 31(3):430–437, 2010.

Cross-Reference

Cardiac Imaging: The REQUISITES, ed 3, pp 324–327.

Comment

Anatomy and Clinical Features

Truncus arteriosus is a cyanotic admixture lesion in which the pulmonary artery and aorta arise from a common trunk. There may be a main pulmonary artery, but in some patients the right and left pulmonary arteries arise separately from the common trunk. A ventricular septal defect is present. The truncal valve usually is tricuspid but can have four or more leaflets. Approximately 30% to 35% of patients have a mirror-image right aortic arch.

Imaging

Radiographs frequently show shunt vascularity, cardiomegaly, and a right-sided aortic arch (Figs. A and B). MRI can be performed to elucidate the anatomy (Fig. C). Velocity-encoded cine MRI can be performed to assess blood flow.

Notes

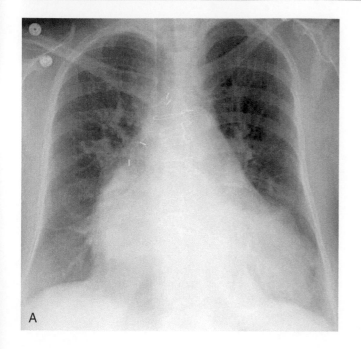

A

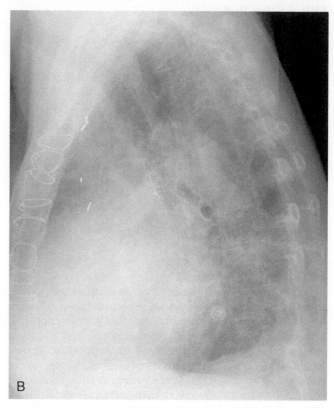

B

History: A patient presents with shortness of breath.

1. What should be included in the differential diagnosis? (Choose all that apply.)
   A. Mitral stenosis
   B. Mitral regurgitation
   C. Mitral valve prolapse
   D. Mitral annular calcification

2. Which of the following diseases is not associated with mitral valve prolapse?
   A. Syphilis
   B. Marfan syndrome
   C. Ehlers-Danlos syndrome
   D. Polycystic kidney disease

3. What is the most common cause of chordae tendineae rupture in this clinical setting?
   A. Elongation of the chordae
   B. Myocardial infarction
   C. Rheumatic heart disease
   D. Iatrogenic

4. What is the most appropriate next step in imaging?
   A. Echocardiography
   B. CT
   C. MRI
   D. Angiography

CASE 132

Mitral Valve Prolapse

1. B and C

2. A

3. A

4. A

References

Bonow RO, Cheitlin MD, Crawford MH, et al: Task Force 3: valvular heart disease, *J Am Coll Cardiol* 45:1334–1340, 2005.

Enriquez-Sarano M, Akins CW, Vahanian A: Mitral regurgitation, *Lancet* 373(9672):1382–1394, 2009.

Cross-Reference

Cardiac Imaging: The REQUISITES, ed 3, pp 192-193.

Comment

Pathology and Etiology

Mitral valve prolapse can involve all components of the mitral apparatus. Mitral valve prolapse has a 5% incidence in the general population. In Marfan syndrome, congenital prolapse occurs in the mitral and tricuspid valves because the valve leaflets are redundant. If prolapse is mild, the heart may be normal. More severe prolapse may result in severe regurgitation, subacute bacterial endocarditis, chest pain, or rarely death. Geometric distortion of the left ventricle can cause moderate mitral valve prolapse.

Imaging Findings

Findings of mitral valve prolapse on chest radiograph are similar to findings of mitral regurgitation from other causes: enlargement of the left atrium and ventricle (Figs. A and B). Mitral valve prolapse can be identified on echocardiography, and echocardiography can be used to grade the severity of prolapse and the presence and degree of regurgitation. Although angiography is not commonly performed for diagnosis, the angiographic hallmark of mitral valve prolapse is the passage of the leaflets behind the plane of the anulus into the left atrium.

Notes

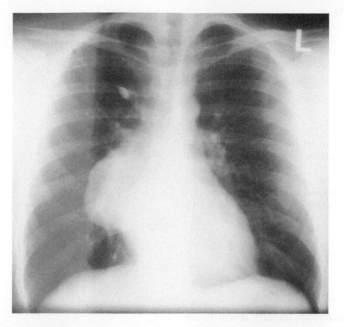

History: No patient history is available.

1. What should be included in the differential
   diagnosis? (Choose all that apply.)
   A. Lymphadenopathy
   B. Bronchogenic cyst
   C. Aortic aneurysm
   D. Sinus of Valsalva aneurysm

2. What is the most common cause of a discrete sinus
   of Valsalva aneurysm?
   A. Atherosclerosis
   B. Syphilis
   C. Weakness at the junction of the aorta and valve
   D. Rheumatic heart disease

3. What valvular lesion is most commonly associated
   with a sinus of Valsalva aneurysm?
   A. Aortic regurgitation
   B. Aortic stenosis
   C. Bicuspid aortic valve
   D. Quadricuspid aortic valve

4. Which type of ventricular septal defect (VSD)
   is associated with a discrete sinus of
   Valsalva aneurysm?
   A. Muscular
   B. Perimembranous
   C. Atrioventricular septal
   D. Supracristal

Sinus of Valsalva Aneurysm

1. A, B, C, and D

2. C

3. B

4. D

References

Hoey ET, Kanagasingam A, Sivananthan MU: Sinus of Valsalva aneurysms: assessment with cardiovascular MRI, *AJR Am J Roentgenol* 194(6):W495-W504, 2010.

Moustafa S, Mookadam F, Cooper L, et al: Sinus of Valsalva aneurysms—47 years of a single center experience and systematic overview of published reports, *Am J Cardiol* 99(8):1159-1164, 2007.

Cross-Reference

Cardiac Imaging: The REQUISITES, ed 3, pp 389-392.

Comment

Etiology and Pathology

Discrete sinus of Valsalva aneurysms usually result from congenital weakness at the junction of the aortic media and the anulus fibrosus of the valve. These aneurysms most frequently arise from the right coronary or noncoronary sinuses. Aneurysms of the right coronary sinus rupture into the right atrium or ventricle, and aneurysms of the noncoronary sinus rupture into the right atrium. Sinus of Valsalva aneurysms are associated with aortic regurgitation. They can occur in patients who have a supracristal VSD.

Imaging

Chest radiograph may be normal or may show a mass arising from the right side of the mediastinum (Figure). On cross-sectional imaging examinations, a discrete sinus of Valsalva aneurysm appears as a focal dilation of one sinus of Valsalva, in contrast to the generalized aortic root dilation seen in annuloaortic ectasia.

Notes

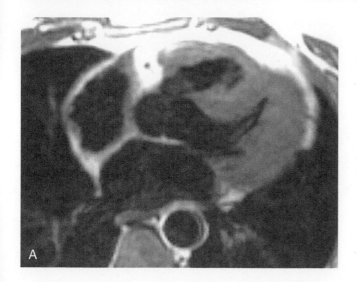

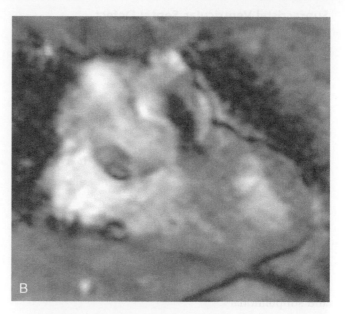

History: An acyanotic patient presents with a murmur.

1. What should be included in the differential diagnosis based on the history? (Choose all that apply.)
   A. Atrial septal defect
   B. Ventricular septal defect (VSD)
   C. Patent ductus arteriosus
   D. Transposition of the great arteries

2. Which type of VSD is depicted by the images?
   A. Muscular
   B. Perimembranous
   C. Atrioventricular septal
   D. Supracristal

3. In Fig. B, what does the black jet indicate?
   A. Left-to-right shunt
   B. Right-to-left shunt
   C. Aortic regurgitation
   D. Aortic stenosis

4. Which abnormality is not associated with a supracristal VSD?
   A. Aortic regurgitation
   B. Aortic stenosis
   C. Sinus of Valsalva aneurysm
   D. Sinus of Valsalva prolapse

Supracristal Ventricular Septal Defect

1. A, B, and C

2. D

3. A

4. B

Reference

Bremerich J, Reddy GP, Higgins CB: MRI of supracristal ventricular septal defects, *J Comput Assist Tomogr* 23(1):13-15, 1999.

Cross-Reference

Cardiac Imaging: The REQUISITES, ed 3, p 60.

Comment

Description of Anomaly

A supracristal VSD is also known as a doubly committed subarterial defect because its location is both subaortic and subpulmonary.

Imaging

Echocardiography is the primary imaging modality for the evaluation of intracardiac shunts. However, because of the location of a supracristal VSD, it may be difficult to assess with echocardiography. MRI demonstrates the characteristic appearance of a connection between the aortic root and right ventricular outflow tract (Fig. A). Steady-state free precession cine images can demonstrate a spin dephasing artifact (black flow jet) directed across the VSD into the pulmonary outflow tract, indicating a left-to-right shunt (Fig. B).

Notes

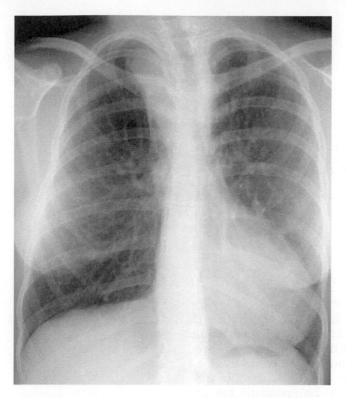

History: A patient presents with a pulsatile supraclavicular mass.

1. What should be included in the differential diagnosis? (Choose all that apply.)
   A. Aneurysm of right aortic arch
   B. Cervical aortic arch
   C. Right subclavian artery aneurysm
   D. Lymphadenopathy

2. Which pharyngeal arch forms the normal aortic arch?
   A. Third
   B. Fourth
   C. Fifth
   D. Sixth

3. Which anomaly can be formed from the right third pharyngeal arch?
   A. Cervical arch
   B. Mirror-image right arch
   C. Left arch with aberrant right subclavian artery
   D. Double aortic arch

4. Which of the following is the least appropriate next step in evaluation?
   A. Percutaneous biopsy
   B. MRI
   C. CT
   D. Echocardiography

CASE 135

Cervical Aortic Arch

1. A, B, and C

2. B

3. A

4. A

References

Caputo S, Villanacci R, Ciampi Q, et al: Cervical aortic arch: echocardiographic and three-dimensional computed tomography view, *Echocardiography* 27(4):E44–E45, 2010.

Poellinger A, Lembcke AE, Elgeti T, et al: Images in cardiovascular medicine. The cervical aortic arch: a rare vascular anomaly, *Circulation* 117(20):2716–2717, 2008.

Cross-Reference

Cardiac Imaging: The REQUISITES, ed 3, p 427.

Comment

Etiology and Clinical Features

Cervical aortic arch is a rare anomaly in which the arch arises from the primitive third arch instead of the fourth. It may be more common on the right side. It has been reported that the ipsilateral internal and external carotid and vertebral arteries arise directly from the arch. Cervical aortic arch is usually asymptomatic but can manifest as a pulsatile mass in the supraclavicular fossa or neck, with obstruction secondary to kinking, or as an aneurysm.

Imaging and Diagnosis

Diagnosis is based on the presence of the aortic arch near the base of the neck (Figure). Some authors state that the diagnosis depends on the finding of separate origins of the internal and external carotid arteries directly from the arch. MRI and CT readily delineate the anatomy.

Notes

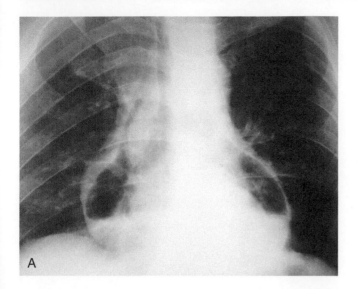

A

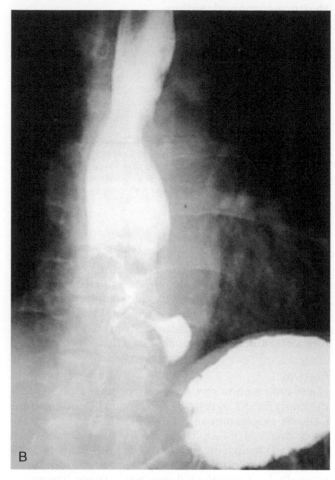

B

History: A patient presents with fever and chest pain.

1. What etiologies can cause the finding seen in Fig. A? (Choose all that apply.)
   A. Trauma
   B. Pericardiocentesis
   C. Barotrauma
   D. Malignant tumor

2. What finding is seen on the upper gastrointestinal (GI) examination (Fig. B)?
   A. Achalasia
   B. Esophageal perforation
   C. Esophageal mass
   D. Esophageal diverticulum

3. In the absence of a history of instrumentation, what is the most likely cause of the finding in Fig. A?
   A. Trauma
   B. Fistula with esophagus
   C. Fistula with bronchus
   D. Fistula with aorta

4. What is the most likely cause of the patient's fever?
   A. Aspiration
   B. Pneumonia
   C. Abscess
   D. Pericarditis

CASE 136

Hydropneumopericardium

1. A, B, C, and D

2. C

3. B

4. D

References

Kaufman J, Thongsuwan N, Stern E, et al: Esophageal-pericardial fistula with purulent pericarditis secondary to esophageal carcinoma presenting with tamponade, *Ann Thorac Surg* 75(1):288–289, 2003.

Meltzer P, Elkayam U, Parsons K, et al: Esophageal-pericardial fistula presenting as pericarditis, *Am Heart J* 105(1):148–150, 1983.

Comment

Etiology

Hydropneumopericardium usually occurs after pericardiocentesis or placement of a pericardial drain. Other causes, such as a fistula, are rare. Tumors that invade the pericardium include breast carcinoma, lung carcinoma, lymphoma, and esophageal carcinoma. Patients with a malignant esophageal-pericardial fistula usually have a diagnosis of metastatic cancer elsewhere in the body.

Imaging

Chest radiography can demonstrate hydropneumopericardium (Fig. A), as can CT, MRI, and echocardiography. Contrast esophagram or endoscopy is helpful in confirming a diagnosis of esophageal carcinoma in patients with suspected malignant fistulae (Fig. B). Patients with malignant or nonmalignant esophageal-pericardial fistula generally have an infected pericardial space. Treatment of a malignant esophageal-pericardial fistula generally requires open drainage and debridement followed by endoscopic placement of an esophageal stent. Percutaneous drainage procedures are generally inadequate as there are often extensive adhesions. Nonmalignant fistulas should ideally be surgically excised or ablated.

Notes

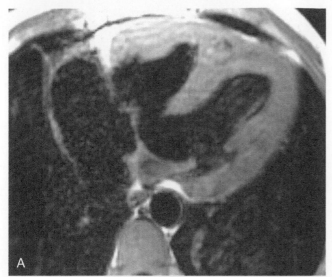

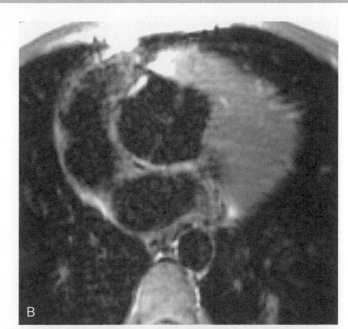

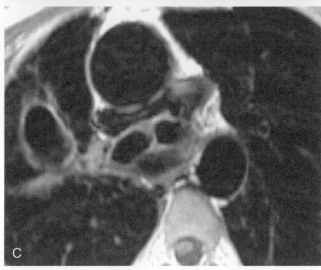

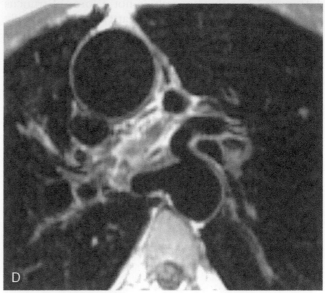

History: A patient has dyspnea on exertion.

1. What findings are seen? (Choose all that apply.)
   A. Right ventricular hypertrophy
   B. Overriding aorta
   C. Pulmonary infundibular stenosis
   D. Ventricular septal defect (VSD)

2. What is the most likely diagnosis?
   A. Atrioventricular septal defect
   B. Tetralogy of Fallot
   C. Transposition of the great arteries.
   D. Pulmonary atresia with VSD

3. How do the lungs receive blood?
   A. Aorta-to-pulmonary artery collaterals
   B. Bronchial arteries
   C. Retrograde flow through pulmonary veins
   D. Arteriovenous malformations.

4. What imaging sequence is depicted?
   A. Inversion recovery
   B. Double inversion recovery
   C. Triple inversion recovery
   D. Delayed enhancement inversion recovery

Pulmonary Atresia with Ventricular Septal Defect

1. A, B, and D

2. D

3. A

4. B

Reference

Reddy GP, Higgins CB: Magnetic resonance imaging of congenital heart disease: evaluation of morphology and function, *Semin Roentgenol* 38(4):342-351, 2003.

Cross-Reference

Cardiac Imaging: The REQUISITES, ed 3, pp 362-363.

Comment

Anomalies of Tetralogy of Fallot

Pulmonary atresia with VSD is a severe variant of tetralogy of Fallot. In the past, it was sometimes called "pseudotruncus," but this anomaly is not a form of truncus arteriosus. The central pulmonary arteries are frequently hypoplastic, and the peripheral pulmonary arteries are often stenotic.

MRI

MRI is optimal for assessing the pulmonary arteries because it evaluates supracardiac structures more readily than echocardiography. Also, MRI does not rely on contrast enhancement to show the vessels, as does cineangiography (Figs. A-D); this is especially useful because the pulmonary arteries usually do not opacify well in the presence of pulmonary atresia.

Notes

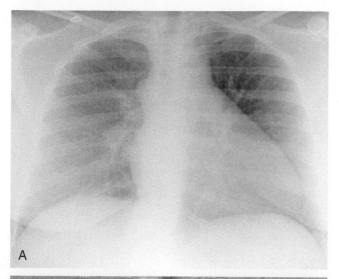

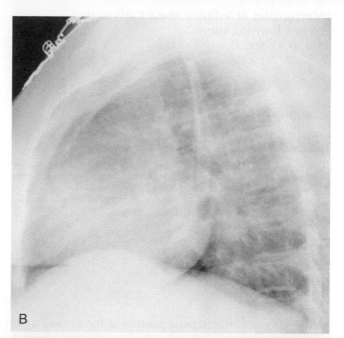

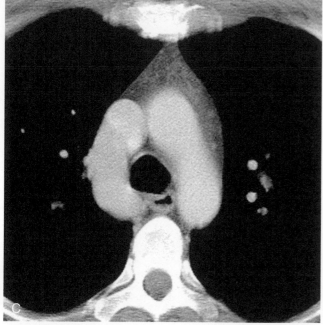

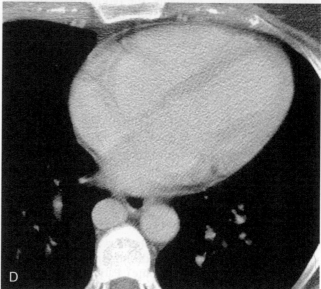

History: No patient history is available.

1. What should be included in the differential diagnosis for dilation of the azygos vein? (Choose all that apply.)
   A. Congestive heart failure
   B. Interruption of inferior vena cava
   C. Constrictive pericarditis
   D. Superior vena cava obstruction

2. What is the most likely diagnosis?
   A. Congestive heart failure
   B. Interruption of inferior vena cava
   C. Constrictive pericarditis
   D. Superior vena cava obstruction

3. Which complex of anomalies is associated with this finding?
   A. Polysplenia
   B. Asplenia
   C. Situs inversus totalis
   D. Situs solitus with levocardia

4. The polysplenia syndrome is highly associated with all of the following features except:
   A. Bilateral left-sidedness
   B. Complex congenital heart disease
   C. Multiple spleens
   D. Common atrium

CASE 138

Interruption of Inferior Vena Cava with Azygos Continuation

1. A, B, C, and D

2. B

3. A

4. B

References

Bass JE, Redwine MD, Kramer LA, et al: Spectrum of congenital anomalies of the inferior vena cava: cross-sectional imaging findings, *Radiographics* 20(3):639–652, 2000.

Jelinek JS, Stuart PL, Done SL, et al: MRI of polysplenia syndrome, *Magn Reson Imaging* 7(6):681–686, 1989.

Cross-Reference

Cardiac Imaging: The REQUISITES, ed 3, pp 307–309.

Comment

Anatomy

In this anomaly, the hepatic portion of the inferior vena cava is interrupted. Typically, the blood passes through collateral channels to enter the azygos or hemiazygos vein. The hepatic veins drain separately into the right atrium. The anomaly may be isolated, as in this case, or it may be associated with polysplenia syndrome which is a type of heterotaxia.

Imaging

Radiography typically demonstrates marked enlargement of the azygos vein (Fig. A). The lateral view may show no inferior vena cava shadow just above the diaphragm (Fig. B). CT and MRI can be performed to evaluate the vascular anatomy and to identify any associated anomalies (Figs. C and D).

Heterotaxia Syndromes

There are two types of heterotaxia syndromes: bilateral right-sidedness (asplenia syndrome) and bilateral left-sidedness (polysplenia syndrome). Patients with asplenia syndrome generally present early in life with cyanosis and complex congenital heart disease (e.g., transposition of the great arteries, double outlet right ventricle, common atrioventricular valve). Patients with polysplenia syndrome present later in life with less severe congenital heart defects (e.g., atrial septal defect, partial anomalous pulmonary venous connection). More than 70% of all patients with polysplenia have either azygos or hemiazygos continuation of the IVC.

Notes

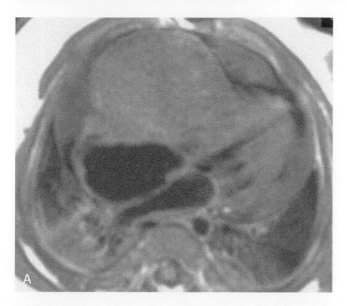

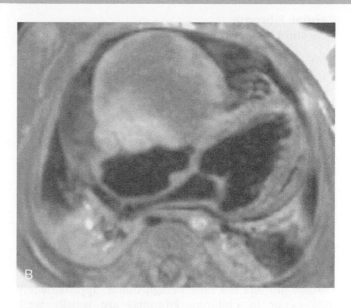

History: An infant presents with vomiting and dehydration.

1. What should be included in the differential diagnosis? (Choose all that apply.)
   A. Rhabdomyoma
   B. Lipoma
   C. Myxoma
   D. Fibroma

2. What is the most common mass in the heart?
   A. Thrombus
   B. Myxoma
   C. Metastasis
   D. Angiosarcoma

3. Which chamber is involved?
   A. Left atrium
   B. Left ventricle
   C. Right atrium
   D. Right ventricle

4. What is the most likely diagnosis?
   A. Rhabdomyoma
   B. Lipoma
   C. Myxoma
   D. Fibroma

Cardiac Fibroma

1. A and D

2. A

3. D

4. D

Reference

Fujita N, Caputo GR, Higgins CB: Diagnosis and characterization of intracardiac masses by magnetic resonance imaging, *Am J Card Imaging* 8(1):69–80, 1994.

Cross-Reference

Cardiac Imaging: The REQUISITES, ed 3, p 278.

Comment

Clinical Information and Histology

Cardiac fibroma is a rare, benign tumor; approximately 90% occur in children. Fibromas are usually well-marginated masses that are mainly composed of spindle cells and intervening collagen. Microscopic calcification is present in approximately half of these tumors.

MRI and Diagnostic Features

MRI demonstrates tumor size and location and cardiac function (Fig. A). Contrast-enhanced MRI can delineate tumor margins and extension and involvement of adjacent structures. However, the presence of enhancement is not reliable for determination of malignancy. Features that suggest a primary malignant cardiac tumor include invasiveness, extension outside the heart, involvement of more than one chamber, central necrosis or cavitation, and large pericardial effusion. Absence of these findings indicates benignancy. The appearance of fibroma is variable on spin echo T1-weighted images and cine MRI. Because fibroma is often isointense to myocardium, the administration of a contrast agent may be necessary to define the extent of a tumor. Fibromas have been reported to show irregular peripheral enhancement or heterogeneous enhancement with dark areas corresponding to calcification (Fig. B). Because gadolinium chelate contrast agent equilibrates rapidly into the extracellular space, the peripheral enhancement pattern indicates poor vascularization of the central fibrous tissue. The periphery of the mass is better vascularized and has a larger extracellular space. Because this enhancement pattern is comparable to that of a fast-growing tumor with central necrosis, it is not diagnostic of a fibroma. Definitive diagnosis requires endomyocardial or open biopsy, but MRI can be used to suggest the diagnosis of fibroma. Surgical resection is performed if the mass causes hemodynamic compromise.

Notes

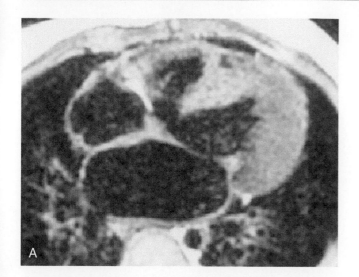

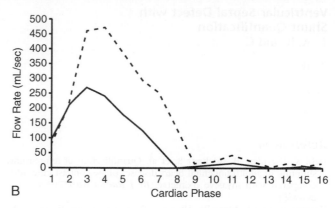

History: An acyanotic patient presents with a murmur.

1. What should be included in the differential diagnosis based on the history? (Choose all that apply.)
   A. Atrial septal defect
   B. Ventricular septal defect (VSD)
   C. Patent ductus arteriosus
   D. Transposition of the great arteries

2. What is the diagnosis?
   A. Atrial septal defect
   B. VSD
   C. Patent ductus arteriosus
   D. Transposition of the great arteries

3. What does the graph (Fig. B) represent?
   A. Pulmonary regurgitation
   B. Aortic stenosis
   C. Collateral circulation
   D. Pulmonary-to-systemic flow ratio

4. What is the interpretation of greater pulmonary blood flow (dashed line) compared with systemic flow (solid line)?
   A. Left-to-right shunt
   B. Right-to-left shunt
   C. Pulmonary hypertension
   D. Eisenmenger syndrome

CASE 140

Ventricular Septal Defect with Shunt Quantification

1. A, B, and C

2. B

3. D

4. A

References

Debl K, Djavidani B, Buchner S, et al: Quantification of left-to-right shunting in adult congenital heart disease: phase-contrast cine MRI compared with invasive oximetry, *Br J Radiol* 82(977):386–391, 2009.

Varaprasathan GA, Araoz PA, Higgins CB, et al: Quantification of flow dynamics in congenital heart disease: applications of velocity-encoded cine MR imaging, *Radiographics* 22(4):895–905; discussion 905–906, 2002.

Wang ZJ, Reddy GP, Gotway MB, et al: Cardiovascular shunts: MR imaging evaluation, *Radiographics* 23(Spec No):S181–S194, 2003.

Cross-Reference

Cardiac Imaging: The REQUISITES, ed 3, pp 72, 340–342.

Comment

Echocardiography

Echocardiography is the mainstay of imaging evaluation of cardiac shunts. Echocardiography can be used to depict the anatomy and assess the degree of shunting.

MRI

MRI has a key role in the assessment of lesions such as supracristal VSD and partial anomalous pulmonary venous return, for which echocardiographic evaluation may be limited (Fig. A). MRI also has an important role in shunt quantification. Velocity-encoded cine MRI can be used to quantify intracardiac shunts with a great degree of accuracy and reproducibility. Velocity-encoded cine MRI is used to measure blood flow in the pulmonary artery (pulmonary flow) and in the ascending aorta (systemic flow). Flow curves are obtained (Fig. B), and the curves are integrated to obtain flow per unit time. In the normal individual, the pulmonary-to-systemic flow ratio is 1:1. However, in a patient with a left-to-right shunt, the ratio is greater than 1. Operative repair may be beneficial when the flow ratio exceeds 1.7:1.

Notes

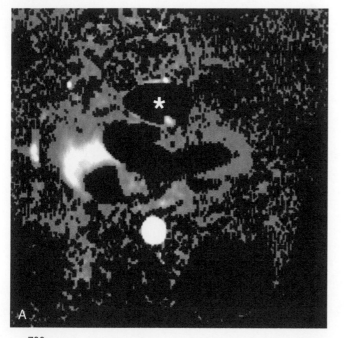

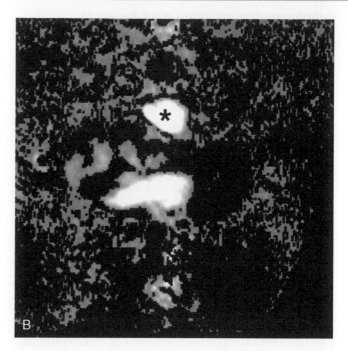

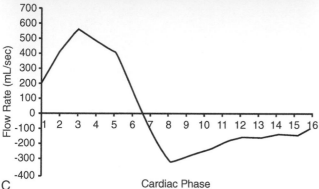

History: A patient presents with dyspnea and murmur after repair of tetralogy of Fallot.

1. What complications can occur after repair of tetralogy of Fallot? (Choose all that apply.)
   A. Right ventricular enlargement
   B. Right ventricular patch aneurysm
   C. Pulmonary stenosis
   D. Pulmonary regurgitation

2. What structure is indicated by the asterisk (Figs. A and B)?
   A. Pulmonary artery
   B. Aorta
   C. Right ventricle
   D. Left ventricle

3. What complication is depicted by the images (Figs. A-C)?
   A. Right ventricular enlargement
   B. Right ventricular patch aneurysm.
   C. Pulmonary stenosis
   D. Pulmonary regurgitation

4. What MRI sequence was used to derive the flow curve?
   A. Steady-state free precession
   B. Velocity-encoded cine MRI
   C. Late gadolinium enhancement inversion recovery
   D. Myocardial tagging

Pulmonary Regurgitation after Repair of Tetralogy of Fallot

1. A, B, and D

2. A

3. D

4. B

Reference

Varaprasathan GA, Araoz PA, Higgins CB, et al: Quantification of flow dynamics in congenital heart disease: applications of velocity-encoded cine MR imaging, *Radiographics* 22(4):895–905; discussion 905–906, 2002.

Cross-Reference

Cardiac Imaging: The REQUISITES, ed 3, pp 72, 363–367.

Comment

Repair of Tetralogy of Fallot

Patients with tetralogy of Fallot typically undergo repair during infancy or early childhood. Frequently, pulmonary infundibular stenosis is relieved by right ventriculoplasty. This procedure can cause long-term pulmonary valve insufficiency. Patients with pulmonary regurgitation may require replacement of the valve.

MRI

Velocity-encoded cine phase contrast images can be used to quantify regurgitation in the postoperative setting (Figs. A-C). MRI is an ideal method to evaluate pulmonary regurgitation because this modality is noninvasive, does not require ionizing radiation, evaluates the right ventricle more readily than echocardiography, and can accurately quantify pulmonary regurgitation and right ventricular volume. Cine MRI is employed for the quantitative appraisal of right ventricular function after surgery.

Notes

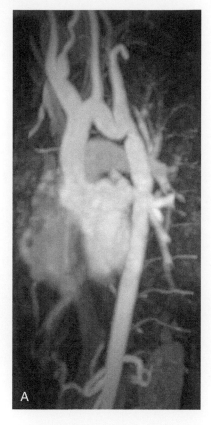

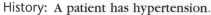

A

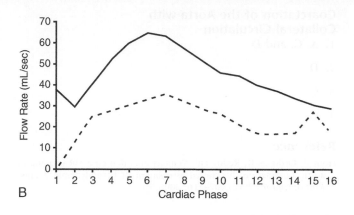

B

History: A patient has hypertension.

1. How can the pressure gradient be measured in coarctation of the aorta? (Choose all that apply.)
   A. Echocardiography
   B. CT
   C. MRI
   D. Angiography

2. Which method can be used to measure collateral blood flow in coarctation of the aorta?
   A. Transthoracic echocardiography
   B. Transesophageal echocardiography
   C. CT
   D. MRI

3. What does the graph (Fig. B) represent?
   A. Peak velocity across the coarctation
   B. Pressure gradient
   C. Collateral circulation
   D. Pulmonary-to-systemic flow ratio

4. In a young adult, what is the most appropriate management?
   A. No treatment
   B. Antihypertensive medication
   C. Angioplasty and stent
   D. Surgery

Coarctation of the Aorta with Collateral Circulation

1. A, C, and D

2. D

3. C

4. C

Reference

Hom JJ, Ordovas K, Reddy GP: Velocity-encoded cine MR imaging in aortic coarctation: functional assessment of hemodynamic events, *Radiographics* 28(2):407–416, 2008.

Cross-Reference

Cardiac Imaging: The REQUISITES, ed 3, pp 72, 420.

Comment

Clinical Features

Congenital coarctation is most commonly discrete and juxtaductal in location (Fig. A). Hypertension is a common finding.

Measurement of Collateral Circulation

Velocity-encoded cine MRI is the only noninvasive method that can accurately quantify collateral circulation in coarctation of the aorta (Fig. B). In normal individuals, flow in the distal thoracic aorta is slightly lower than in the proximal descending aorta because the intercostal arteries and other aortic branches take blood away from the aorta. However, in a patient with a functionally significant coarctation, collateral vessels bring blood into the descending thoracic aorta, and the distal flow is greater than the proximal flow. The presence of collateral flow shows that the lesion is hemodynamically significant, even in the absence of visible collateral vessels.

Notes

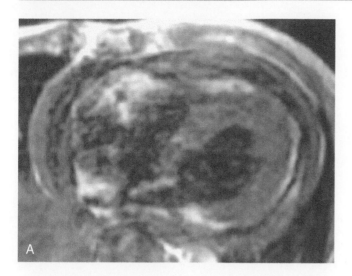

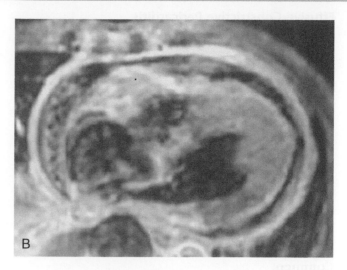

History: A patient presents with dyspnea on exertion, pleural effusions, and ascites.

1. What pericardial findings are seen? (Choose all that apply.)
   A. Effusion
   B. Thickening
   C. Calcification
   D. Enhancement

2. What is the most likely etiology?
   A. Fungal infection
   B. Bacterial infection
   C. Viral infection
   D. Tuberculosis

3. Given the symptoms and MRI images, what is the most likely diagnosis?
   A. Acute pericarditis
   B. Tamponade
   C. Effusive constrictive pericarditis
   D. Tumor

4. Which of the following is NOT an MRI imaging finding seen in constrictive pericarditis?
   A. Pericardial thickening greater than 4 mm
   B. Diffuse subendocardial late gadolinium enhancement
   C. Septal bounce
   D. Right atrial and inferior vena cava dilation

Effusive Constrictive Pericarditis

1. A, B, and D

2. D

3. C

4. B

References

Syed FF, Ntsekhe M, Mayosi BM, et al: Effusive-constrictive pericarditis, *Heart Fail Rev* 2012 Mar 16 [Epub ahead of print].

Wang ZJ, Reddy GP, Gotway MB, et al: CT and MR imaging of pericardial disease, *Radiographics* 23(Spec No):S167–S180, 2003.

Cross-Reference

Cardiac Imaging: The REQUISITES, ed 3, p 269.

Comment

Etiology and Characteristic Features

Effusive constrictive pericarditis is most commonly caused by tuberculosis. Pericardial effusions and pericardial thickening are characteristic. In the setting of constrictive/restrictive physiology, the diagnosis is effusive constrictive pericarditis. Pericardiocentesis can relieve the acute illness and can aid in diagnosis, but chronic constrictive pericarditis can develop.

Imaging

CT or MRI can show a complex pericardial effusion and pericardial thickening and enhancement (Figs. A and B). If the patient has symptoms of constriction, the diagnosis of effusive constrictive pericarditis can be made.

Notes

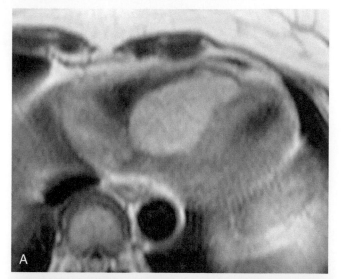

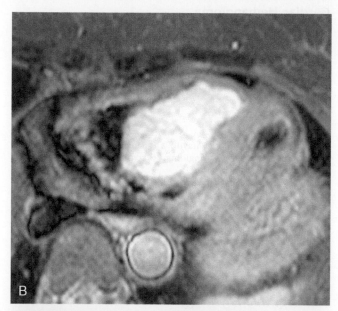

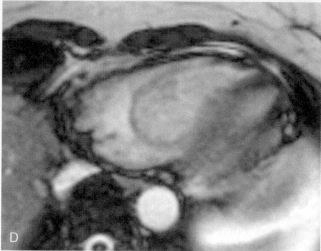

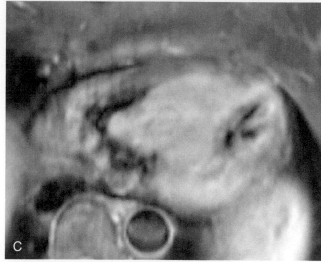

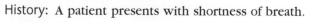

History: A patient presents with shortness of breath.

1. What features are characteristic of a malignant cardiac tumor? (Choose all that apply.)
   A. Infiltrative appearance
   B. Involvement of two or more chambers
   C. Extension outside of the heart
   D. Central necrosis

2. What is the most common tumor in the heart?
   A. Fibroma
   B. Myxoma
   C. Metastasis
   D. Hemangioma

3. Which chamber is involved?
   A. Left atrium
   B. Left ventricle
   C. Right atrium
   D. Right ventricle

4. What is the most likely diagnosis?
   A. Hemangioma
   B. Lipoma
   C. Myxoma
   D. Fibroma

CASE 144

Cardiac Hemangioma

1. A, B, C, and D

2. C

3. D

4. A

References

Moniotte S, Geva T, Perez-Atayde A, et al: Images in cardiovascular medicine. Cardiac hemangioma, *Circulation* 112(8):E103–E104, 2005.

Randhawa K, Ganeshan A, Hoey ET: Magnetic resonance imaging of cardiac tumors: part 1, sequences, protocols, and benign tumors, *Curr Probl Diagn Radiol* 40(4):158–168, 2011.

Cross-Reference

Cardiac Imaging: The REQUISITES, ed 3, p 280.

Comment

Histology and Physiology

Hemangiomas are benign proliferations of endothelial cells and vessels. These masses can be classified as a cavernous, a capillary, or an arteriovenous subtype, depending on the dominant vascular channel. Hemangiomas can contain calcification, fat, and fibrous tissue. Cardiac hemangiomas are rare and can be intramural or within a chamber.

Clinical symptoms and signs include dyspnea on exertion, arrhythmia, angina, and right heart failure. Right ventricular outflow obstruction is the usual cause of dyspnea in patients with hemangioma.

CT and MRI

CT can be used to delineate the location, size, and extent of the mass. On CT, a hemangioma is typically heterogeneous and often demonstrates areas of calcification. Iodinated contrast agent is useful to demonstrate marked enhancement of this vascular mass. MRI can provide optimal evaluation of a cardiac mass (Figs. A-D). Hemangiomas demonstrate low to intermediate signal intensity on T1-weighted images and high signal intensity on T2-weighted images, but occasionally the mass also shows high signal intensity on T1-weighted images. When a mass demonstrates high signal intensity on T1-weighted images, it is important to consider the diagnoses of lipoma and melanoma in addition to hemangioma. Hemangiomas do not lose signal with fat suppression techniques, allowing differentiation from lipomas. Melanoma metastases and other malignant tumors are infiltrative, in contrast to a hemangioma.

Notes

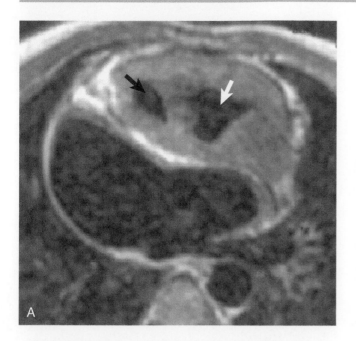

A

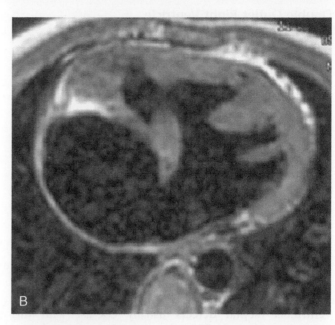

B

History: A patient presents with cyanosis.

1. What should be included in the differential diagnosis in a patient with cyanosis and increased pulmonary vascularity? (Choose all that apply.)
   A. Transposition of the great arteries
   B. Total anomalous pulmonary venous connection
   C. Double-outlet right ventricle
   D. Truncus arteriosus

2. What structure is indicated by the black arrow in Fig. A?
   A. Pulmonary artery
   B. Ascending aorta
   C. Descending aorta
   D. Superior vena cava

3. What structure is indicated by the white arrow in Fig. A?
   A. Pulmonary artery
   B. Ascending aorta
   C. Descending aorta
   D. Superior vena cava

4. What is the most likely diagnosis?
   A. Transposition of the great arteries
   B. Total anomalous pulmonary venous connection
   C. Double-outlet right ventricle
   D. Truncus arteriosus

CASE 145

Double-Outlet Right Ventricle

1. A, B, C, and D

2. B

3. A

4. C

Reference

Reddy GP, Higgins CB: Magnetic resonance imaging of congenital heart disease: evaluation of morphology and function, *Semin Roentgenol* 38(4):342-351, 2003.

Cross-Reference

Cardiac Imaging: The REQUISITES, ed 3, pp 322-324.

Comment

Anatomy and Associated Anomalies

Double-outlet right ventricle is a rare admixture lesion that causes shunt vascularity and cyanosis. Atrial and ventricular septal defects usually coexist with this anomaly, and about 75% of patients have some degree of pulmonic stenosis or atresia. Several coronary artery anomalies may coexist with double-outlet right ventricle, including anomalous origin of the right coronary artery from the left coronary artery, anomalous origin of the left anterior descending coronary artery from the right coronary artery, and duplication of the left anterior descending coronary artery.

Imaging

Radiographs typically show shunt vascularity and cardiomegaly. The diagnosis is made by ascertaining that both great arteries arise from a muscular infundibulum, indicating a right ventricular origin. In most patients, the aorta is to the right of the main pulmonary artery (so-called D-malposition). The diagnosis can be made with echocardiography in most patients. MRI readily demonstrates the pathologic anatomy and is helpful in making the diagnosis of double-outlet right ventricle (Figs. A and B) in equivocal or confusing cases. MRI also accurately depicts the size and orientation of the ventricular septal defect, which guides surgical management.

Treatment

The major goal of treatment is to restore biventricular function, and surgery is usually performed before the first birthday. The surgical approach varies depending on the orientation of the ventricular septal defect. Complications of surgery include subaortic stenosis, severe pulmonic regurgitation with right ventricular dysfunction, and pulmonic outflow tract obstruction. These complications vary depending on the surgical approach.

Notes

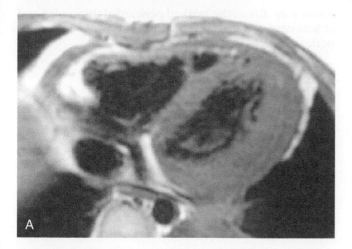

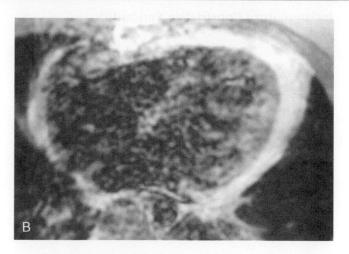

History: A patient presents with fatigue, progressive dyspnea on exertion, and lower extremity swelling after surgical repair of an atrial septal defect.

1. What etiologies can cause this finding? (Choose all that apply.)
   A. Open heart surgery
   B. Radiation therapy
   C. Viral infection
   D. Tuberculosis

2. What is the pericardial abnormality in Fig. A?
   A. Effusion
   B. Thickening
   C. Calcification
   D. Nodularity

3. Given the symptoms and both images, what is the most likely diagnosis?
   A. Acute pericarditis
   B. Inflammatory constrictive pericarditis
   C. Effusive constrictive pericarditis
   D. Tumor

4. What is the most appropriate treatment?
   A. Antibiotics
   B. Pericardial stripping
   C. Pericardiocentesis
   D. Radiation therapy

Inflammatory Constrictive Pericarditis

1. A, B, C, and D

2. B

3. B

4. B

Reference

Wang ZJ, Reddy GP, Gotway MB, et al: CT and MR imaging of pericardial disease, *Radiographics* 23(Spec No):S167–S180, 2003.

Cross-Reference

Cardiac Imaging: The REQUISITES, ed 3, pp 269-271.

Comment

Etiology and Physiology

Constrictive pericarditis occurs when limitation in diastolic ventricular filling leads to equalization of atrial and ventricular pressure, which is known as constrictive/restrictive physiology. Patients have symptoms similar to congestive heart failure. Physical examination may demonstrate the classic Kussmaul sign, which is the paradoxical elevation of jugular venous pressure on inspiration. Causes of constrictive pericarditis include open heart surgery, radiation therapy, uremic pericarditis, viral pericarditis, and tuberculous pericarditis (this is less common in industrialized countries).

Treatment

Constrictive pericarditis and restrictive cardiomyopathy have similar clinical presentations and findings on echocardiography and cardiac catheterization. However, it is important to differentiate between these two diseases because patients with constrictive disease usually benefit from pericardiectomy, whereas patients with restrictive cardiomyopathy have a poor prognosis and must be managed medically or with heart transplantation. Constrictive pericarditis, whether acute or chronic, can be treated by pericardial stripping.

Imaging

In the clinical setting of constrictive/restrictive physiology, pericardial thickening (≥4 mm) as demonstrated on MRI can establish the diagnosis of constrictive pericarditis (Figs. A and B). Pericardial thickening may be diffuse or localized to the right heart or atrioventricular grooves. Diastolic septal dysfunction (septal bounce) on cine MRI is another key finding. Ancillary findings may be present, including dilation of the inferior vena cava, hepatic veins, and right atrium, with a narrow, tubular right ventricle. It is important to remember that pericardial thickening can occur in the absence of constrictive physiology, and not all cases of surgically proven constrictive pericarditis have pericardial thickening. The diagnosis of constrictive pericarditis can be established only in the appropriate clinical setting of constrictive/restrictive physiology. Given the marked pericardial thickening and enhancement, the diagnosis of inflammatory constrictive pericarditis can be established.

Notes

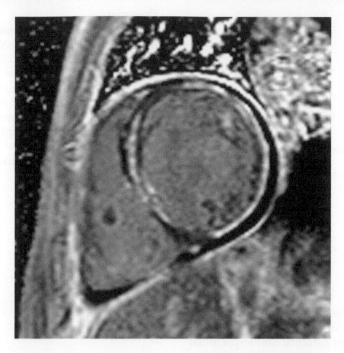

History: A 24-year-old man presents with shortness of breath and chest pain.

1. What should be included in the differential diagnosis? (Choose all that apply.)
   A. Hypertrophic cardiomyopathy
   B. Sarcoidosis
   C. Constrictive pericarditis
   D. Myocarditis

2. What is an appropriate dose of gadolinium chelate contrast agent for late gadolinium enhancement imaging?
   A. 0.01 mmol/kg
   B. 0.05 mmol/kg
   C. 0.15 mmol/kg
   D. 0.5 mmol/kg

3. What is the most likely diagnosis if the patient's chest radiograph was clear and his chest pain started after a viral illness?
   A. Amyloidosis
   B. Myocarditis
   C. Infarction
   D. Sarcoidosis

4. What is an appropriate delay between administration of gadolinium chelate contrast agent and the acquisition of the inversion recovery sequences?
   A. 10 seconds
   B. 2 minutes
   C. 10 minutes
   D. 30 minutes

CASE 147

Acute Myocarditis

1. B and D

2. C

3. B

4. C

References

Feldman AM, McNamara D: Myocarditis, *N Engl J Med* 343(19):1388–1398, 2000.⊙

Ordovas KG, Higgins CB: Delayed contrast enhancement on MR images of myocardium: past, present, future, *Radiology* 261(2):358–374, 2011.⊙

Cross-Reference

Cardiac Imaging: The REQUISITES, ed 3, pp 91–92, 292–294.

Comment

Clinical Features

Myocarditis is the inflammation of myocardial tissue that most commonly follows a viral infection. It is a cause of sudden cardiac death in young patients. Endomyocardial biopsy is considered the gold standard for diagnosis, but it is invasive and may be negative because of sampling error. Myocarditis is usually self-limiting, and supportive therapy may be indicated.

MRI

MRI is often used to diagnose myocarditis. Several MRI sequences can be performed, but the most useful is the inversion recovery late gadolinium enhancement sequence. Late gadolinium enhancement in a nonischemic pattern (typically midmyocardial) supports the diagnosis of myocarditis (Figure). MRI identifies the disease in 30% of patients with chest pain, elevated troponin, and clinically normal coronary arteries. Three findings are assessed to make the diagnosis of myocarditis:

1. T2 hyperintensity (focal or diffuse) indicates inflammation and edema. This is potentially reversible in the setting of no late gadolinium enhancement.

2. Early gadolinium enhancement (focal or diffuse) obtained minutes after gadolinium injection indicates hyperemia and capillary leak.

3. Late gadolinium enhancement that is patchy and does not correspond to a typical vascular distribution indicates irreversible injury with necrosis and fibrosis.

Test sensitivity and specificity for diagnosing myocarditis increase with more positive findings (i.e., T2 hyperintensity, early gadolinium enhancement, and late gadolinium enhancement).

Prognosis

Late gadolinium enhancement occurring 4 weeks after the acute episode has shown prognostic value in predicting poor functional and clinical outcomes. A reduced ejection fraction and right ventricular involvement are echocardiographic markers of an increased risk for sudden cardiac death and future need for cardiac transplantation. Patients with myocarditis are usually treated supportively with heart failure and arrhythmia management. Immunosuppressive therapy is initiated when it results from an autoimmune disease.

Notes

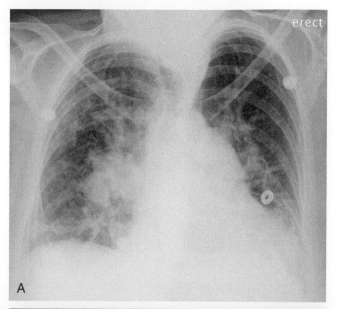

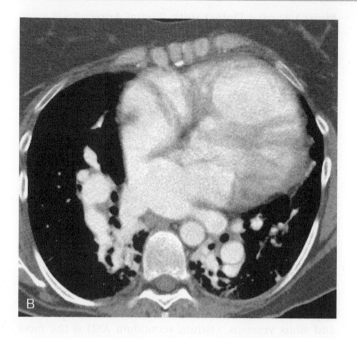

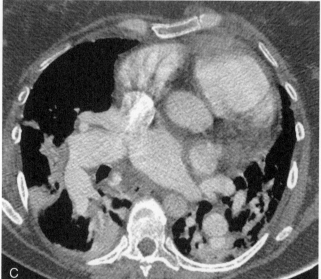

History: An acyanotic patient presents with shortness of breath and murmur.

1. What should be included in the differential diagnosis? (Choose all that apply.)
   A. Ventricular septal defect
   B. Atrial septal defect (ASD)
   C. Partial anomalous pulmonary venous connection (PAPVC)
   D. Tetralogy of Fallot

2. Which septal defect is most commonly associated with PAPVC?
   A. Secundum ASD
   B. Primum ASD
   C. Sinus venosus defect
   D. Ventricular septal defect

3. What type of septal defect is seen in this patient?
   A. Secundum ASD
   B. Primum ASD
   C. Sinus venosus defect
   D. Ventricular septal defect

4. Which of the following most commonly occurs in the setting of long-standing ASD?
   A. Systemic hypertension
   B. Pulmonary hypertension
   C. Paradoxical embolism
   D. Pulmonary embolism

CASE 148

Sinus Venosus Defect with Partial Anomalous Pulmonary Venous Connection

1. A, B, and C

2. C

3. C

4. B

Reference

Higgins CB: Radiography of congenital heart disease. In Webb WR, Higgins CB, editors: *Thoracic imaging: pulmonary and cardiovascular radiology*, ed 2, Philadelphia, 2010, Lippincott Williams & Wilkins.

Cross-Reference

Cardiac Imaging: The REQUISITES, ed 3, pp 335-338.

Comment

Types of ASD

Types of ASD include ostium secundum, ostium primum, and sinus venosus. Ostium secundum ASD is the most common type and is the most frequently diagnosed left-to-right shunt in adult patients. An ostium primum ASD is present in atrioventricular septal defect (formerly known as endocardial cushion defect). A sinus venosus defect (Fig. B) occurs at the lateral superior portion of the ventricular septum, at the posterior wall of the superior vena cava, and is commonly associated with PAPVC. Patients with both PAPVC and ASD can be asymptomatic but may present with dyspnea, exercise intolerance, pulmonary hypertension, or syncope depending on the degree of shunt.

Imaging Findings

Although the chest radiograph may be normal when the shunt is small, pulmonary vascularity is usually increased (shunt vascularity) (Fig. A). PAPVC is another atrial-level shunt that can mimic an ASD physiologically and can appear similar to ASD on a chest radiograph. Echocardiography can delineate the size and location of the ASD. MRI or CT can be performed if echocardiography does not demonstrate a suspected ASD (Fig. B) and can be used to identify anomalous pulmonary veins (Fig. C). MRI can quantify the shunt fraction and helps determine the ideal timing to perform surgery. The indications for surgical correction are symptoms or a large shunt (i.e., pulmonary blood flow twice that of systemic blood flow).

Notes

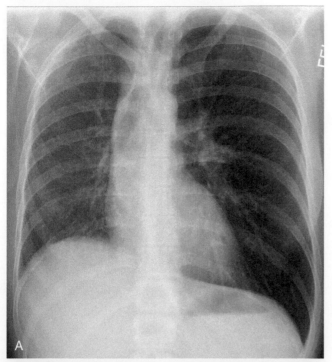

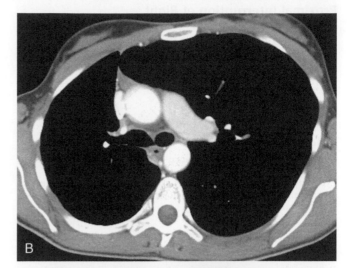

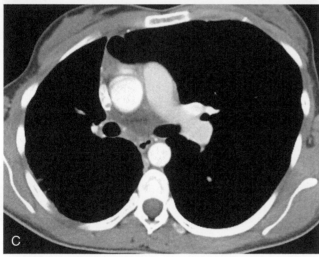

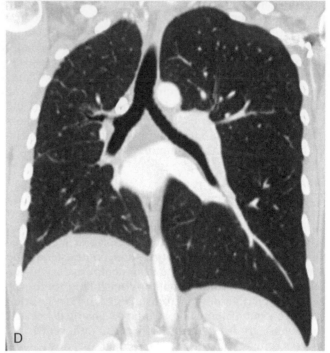

History: A patient presents with dyspnea on exertion.

1. Which abnormalities are seen on the radiograph?
   (Choose all that apply.)
   A. Right lung hypoplasia
   B. Diaphragmatic hernia
   C. Scimitar vein
   D. Diminutive right hilum

2. Which structure is absent on the CT scan?
   A. Aortic arch
   B. Trachea
   C. Esophagus
   D. Right pulmonary artery

3. What is the most likely diagnosis?
   A. Pulmonary sling
   B. Pulmonary atresia
   C. Pulmonic valve stenosis
   D. Proximal interruption of the right
      pulmonary artery

4. How does the right pulmonary artery system
   receive its blood supply?
   A. Reconstitution of the right pulmonary artery
   B. Bronchial arteries
   C. Systemic-to-pulmonary artery collaterals
   D. Pulmonary veins

CASE 149

Proximal Interruption of Right Pulmonary Artery

1. A and D

2. D

3. D

4. C

References

Hernandez RJ: Magnetic resonance imaging of mediastinal vessels, *Magn Reson Imaging Clin N Am* 10(2):237–251, 2002.

Zylak CJ, Eyler WR, Spizarny DL, et al: Developmental lung anomalies in the adult: radiologic-pathologic correlation, *Radiographics* 22(Spec No):S25–S43, 2002.

Comment

Anatomy

Proximal interruption of pulmonary artery, or "absent pulmonary artery," is a rare anomaly that occurs contralateral to the aortic arch. Although the proximal segment of the pulmonary artery is absent, there is a rudimentary artery in the hilum. The affected lung is usually hypoplastic, and it receives blood flow via systemic-to-pulmonary collateral channels arising from the bronchial, intercostal, brachiocephalic, subclavian, and smaller systemic arteries. Interruption of the left pulmonary artery is commonly associated with other congenital heart defects (most commonly tetralogy of Fallot).

Imaging

The diagnosis depends on nonvisualization of the artery on echocardiography, CT scan, or MRI (Figs. B-D). Chest radiographic findings (Fig. A) include a small hemithorax with signs of volume loss (e.g., ipsilateral mediastinal shift, hemidiaphragm elevation, and contralateral lung rotation to the opposite side from compensatory hyperinflation). The ipsilateral hilum is small, and there may be unilateral rib notching from enlarged intercostal arteries. The contralateral hilum appears enlarged because the pulmonary artery receives the entire right ventricular stroke volume. Important differential diagnostic considerations for the radiographic appearance include Swyer-James syndrome (constrictive bronchiolitis from a childhood infection) and pulmonary hypoplasia, such as occurs in scimitar syndrome.

Notes

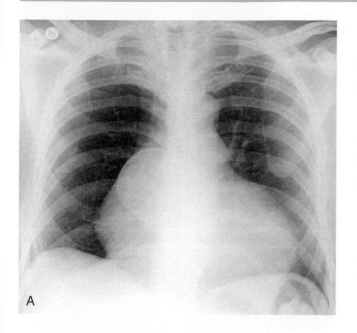

A

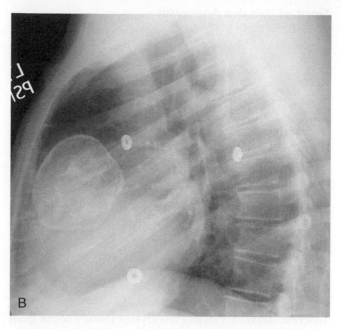

B

History: A patient presents with chest pain.

1. What should be included in the differential diagnosis? (Choose all that apply.)
   A. Sinus of Valsalva aneurysm
   B. Aortic aneurysm
   C. Lymphadenopathy
   D. Bronchogenic cyst

2. What is the most common cause of a discrete sinus of Valsalva aneurysm?
   A. Atherosclerosis
   B. Syphilis
   C. Weakness at the junction of the aorta and valve
   D. Rheumatic heart disease

3. What valvular lesion is most commonly associated with a sinus of Valsalva aneurysm?
   A. Aortic regurgitation
   B. Aortic stenosis
   C. Bicuspid aortic valve
   D. Quadricuspid aortic valve

4. Which type of ventricular septal defect (VSD) is associated with a discrete sinus of Valsalva aneurysm?
   A. Muscular
   B. Perimembranous
   C. Atrioventricular septal
   D. Supracristal

CASE 150

Sinus of Valsalva Aneurysm

1. A, B, C, and D

2. C

3. A

4. D

References

Hoey ET, Kanagasingam A, Sivananthan MU: Sinus of Valsalva aneurysms: assessment with cardiovascular MRI, *AJR Am J Roentgenol* 194(6):W495-W504, 2010.

Moustafa S, Mookadam F, Cooper L, et al: Sinus of Valsalva aneurysms—47 years of a single center experience and systematic overview of published reports, *Am J Cardiol* 99(8):1159-1164, 2007.

Cross-Reference

Cardiac Imaging: The REQUISITES, ed 3, pp 389-392.

Comment

Etiology and Pathology

Discrete sinus of Valsalva aneurysms usually result from congenital weakness at the junction of the aortic media and the annulus fibrosus of the valve. They most frequently arise from the right coronary or noncoronary sinuses. Aneurysms of the right coronary sinus rupture into the right atrium or right ventricle, and aneurysms of the noncoronary sinus rupture into the right atrium. Sinus of Valsalva aneurysms are associated with aortic regurgitation. They can occur in patients who have a supracristal VSD.

Imaging

Chest radiography may be normal or may show a mass arising from the right side of the mediastinum (Figs. A and B). On cross-sectional imaging examinations, a discrete sinus of Valsalva aneurysm manifests as a focal dilation of one sinus of Valsalva, in contrast to the generalized aortic root dilation seen in annuloaortic ectasia. Calcification can be seen in these lesions (Figs. A and B).

Notes

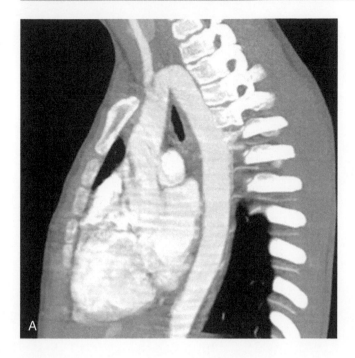

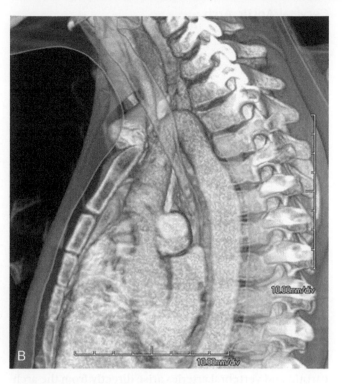

History: An 11-year-old boy presents with a pulsatile mass on the right side at the base of the neck.

1. What abnormalities can cause a pulsatile mass at the base of the neck? (Choose all that apply.)
   A. Lymphadenopathy
   B. Cervical aortic arch
   C. Right subclavian artery aneurysm
   D. Aneurysm of right aortic arch

2. Which pharyngeal arch forms the normal aortic arch?
   A. Third
   B. Fourth
   C. Fifth
   D. Sixth

3. The right third pharyngeal arch can form which anomaly?
   A. Double aortic arch
   B. Cervical arch
   C. Left arch with aberrant right subclavian artery
   D. Mirror-image right arch

4. Based on the CT scan, what is the most likely diagnosis?
   A. Lymphadenopathy
   B. Cervical aortic arch
   C. Right subclavian artery aneurysm
   D. Aneurysm of right aortic arch

Cervical Aortic Arch

1. B, C, and D

2. B

3. B

4. B

References

Caputo S, Villanacci R, Ciampi Q, et al: Cervical aortic arch: echocardiographic and three-dimensional computed tomography view, *Echocardiography* 27(4):E44-E45, 2010.

Poellinger A, Lembcke AE, Elgeti T, et al: Images in cardiovascular medicine. The cervical aortic arch: a rare vascular anomaly, *Circulation* 117(20):2716-2717, 2008.

Cross-Reference

Cardiac Imaging: The REQUISITES, ed 3, p 427.

Comment

Etiology and Clinical Features

Cervical aortic arch is a rare anomaly in which the arch arises from the primitive third arch instead of the fourth arch. It may be more common on the right side. It has been reported that the ipsilateral internal and external carotid and vertebral arteries arise directly from the arch. Cervical aortic arch is usually asymptomatic but can manifest as a pulsatile mass in the supraclavicular fossa or neck, with obstruction from kinking, or as an aneurysm. Other symptoms include stridor, frequent respiratory infections, and dyspnea on exertion. Patients with cervical aortic arch do not require treatment unless there is an aneurysm or respiratory symptoms.

Imaging and Diagnosis

Diagnosis is based on the presence of the aortic arch near the base of the neck. Some authors state that the diagnosis depends on the finding of separate origins of the internal and external carotid arteries directly from the arch. MRI and CT delineate the anatomy (Figs. A and B). A cervical aortic arch extends above the level of the clavicles and manubrium and may extend to the C2 vertebral body.

Notes

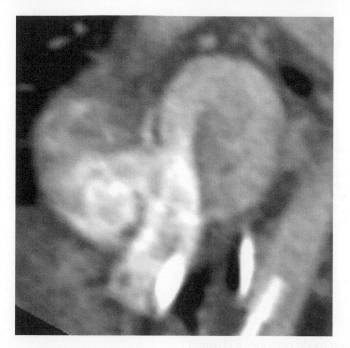

History: A neonate underwent a CT scan performed with contrast agent injection into the umbilical vein catheter.

1. What should be included in the differential diagnosis based on the pattern of chamber opacification? (Choose all that apply.)
   A. Ventricular septal defect
   B. Atrial septal defect
   C. Partial anomalous pulmonary venous connection
   D. Patent foramen ovale

2. Which cardiac chamber should opacify first after contrast agent injection into the umbilical vein catheter?
   A. Left atrium
   B. Left ventricle
   C. Right atrium
   D. Right ventricle

3. What is the purpose of the foramen ovale?
   A. To allow right-to-left shunting in fetal life
   B. To allow left-to-right shunting in fetal life
   C. To allow right-to-left shunting in postnatal life
   D. To allow left-to-right shunting in postnatal life

4. If the foramen ovale remains patent, what is the most significant complication?
   A. Cyanosis
   B. Pulmonary hypertension
   C. Paradoxical embolism
   D. Pulmonary embolism

CASE 152

Patent Foramen Ovale

1. B and D

2. C

3. A

4. C

References

Berko NS, Haramati LB: Simple cardiac shunts in adults, *Semin Roentgenol* 47(3):277-288, 2012.

Kim YJ, Hur J, Shim CY, et al: Patent foramen ovale: diagnosis with multidetector CT—comparison with transesophageal echocardiography, *Radiology* 250(1):61-67, 2009.

Kutty S, Sengupta PP, Khandheria BK: Patent foramen ovale: the known and the to be known, *J Am Coll Cardiol* 59(19):1665-1671, 2012.

Cross-Reference

Cardiac Imaging: The REQUISITES, ed 3, p 335.

Comment

Clinical Features

In fetal life, the patent foramen ovale provides a channel for umbilical vein blood to bypass the lungs and enter the systemic circulation directly. The foramen is covered by a flap that should close after birth. However, the flap does not close in a substantial minority of individuals, and approximately 25% of adults have a patent foramen ovale. The most important complication of this condition is paradoxical embolism, which can result in ischemia or infarction in one or more organs, including the brain. Some patients are treated with a transcatheter septal occluder device.

Imaging Findings

Echocardiography and occasionally CT (Figure) and MRI can demonstrate blood flowing across the foramen ovale. The direction of the shunt can be from left to right in a substantial percentage of people or may reverse (as in the case shown) when right atrial pressure exceeds left atrial pressure as in coughing or with the Valsalva maneuver. The patent foramen ovale typically has a small channel-like configuration on CT or MRI. To make a confident diagnosis on CT, both the channel-like configuration in the interatrial septum and a jet of contrast medium passing between the atria must be observed. The standard reference, transesophageal echocardiography with agitated saline, detects a patent foramen ovale by momentarily seeing microbubbles passing across the interatrial septum into the left atrium during provocative maneuvers. Many clinicians believe that echocardiography may miss a substantial percentage of cases of patent foramen ovale, especially in patients who cannot cooperate with Valsalva instructions.

Notes

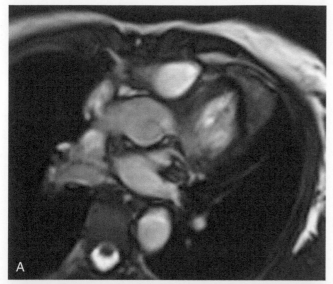

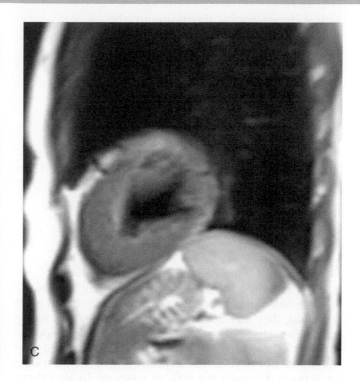

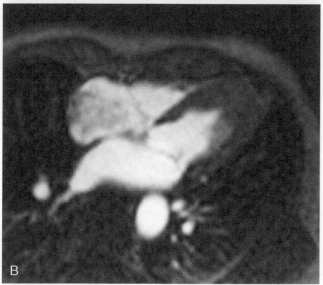

History: A patient is status post left lung transplant.

1. What are possible distributions of hypertrophic cardiomyopathy (HCM)? (Choose all that apply.)
   A. Septal
   B. Concentric
   C. Midventricular
   D. Apical

2. What is the distribution of hypertrophy in this patient?
   A. Septal
   B. Concentric
   C. Midventricular
   D. Apical

3. Which country has the highest prevalence of apical HCM?
   A. United States
   B. South Africa
   C. Japan
   D. Brazil

4. What is the etiology of HCM?
   A. Sarcoidosis
   B. Hypertension
   C. Ischemia
   D. Genetic

Apical Hypertrophic Cardiomyopathy

1. A, B, C, and D

2. D

3. C

4. D

Reference

Harris SR, Glockner J, Misselt AJ, et al: Cardiac MR imaging of nonischemic cardiomyopathies, *Magn Reson Imaging Clin N Am* 16(2):165–183, 2008.

Cross-Reference

Cardiac Imaging: The REQUISITES, ed 3, pp 53, 284–288.

Comment

Etiology and Clinical Features

HCM is inherited as an autosomal dominant trait with variable penetrance. Patients have a variable clinical presentation; they may be asymptomatic, or they may have atrial fibrillation, heart failure, syncope, or sudden cardiac death, which is the leading cause of mortality in these patients. Asymmetric hypertrophy of the ventricular septum accounts for 90% of cases of HCM. Other patterns exhibit a right ventricular, left ventricular, septal, apical, midventricular, or concentric distribution. The apical pattern can account for 25% of patients in Japan, but it is uncommon elsewhere. Patients with heart failure secondary to significant hypertrophy can be treated with myectomy.

Imaging

MRI (Figs. A-C) can provide anatomic and functional information in HCM and can be most useful when the diagnosis is in question, when invasive therapy is being considered, or when clinical concern requires more thorough assessment than provided by echocardiography. MRI can be used to identify the distribution of thickened myocardium and to calculate left ventricular mass. Therapy may depend on the distribution of hypertrophy. MRI also can be used for functional evaluation of left ventricular outflow tract obstruction and myocardial perfusion and viability.

Notes

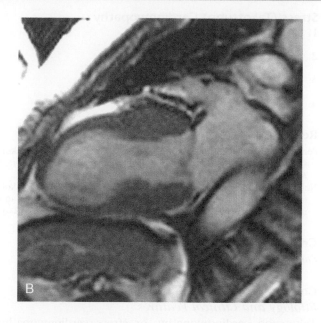

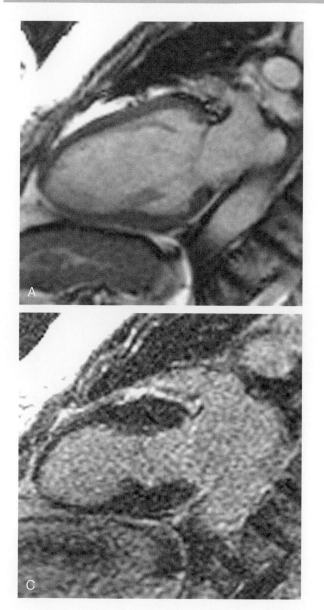

History: A 72-year-old woman with a history of systemic hypertension and seizure disorder presents with chest pressure, racing heart, and sensation of being scared.

1. What should be included in the differential diagnosis based on the history and the steady-state free precession (SSFP) images (Figs. A and B)? (Choose all that apply.)
A. Myocardial infarction
B. Noncompaction cardiomyopathy
C. Takotsubo cardiomyopathy
D. Hypertrophic cardiomyopathy

2. What does the late gadolinium enhancement image show?
A. No late gadolinium enhancement
B. Midmyocardial late gadolinium enhancement
C. Subendocardial late gadolinium enhancement
D. Transmural late gadolinium enhancement

3. Based on the history and the figures, what is the most likely diagnosis?
A. Myocardial infarction
B. Noncompaction cardiomyopathy
C. Takotsubo cardiomyopathy
D. Hypertrophic cardiomyopathy

4. Which imaging plane was used in these sequences?
A. Short axis
B. Vertical long axis
C. Horizontal long axis
D. Left ventricular outflow tract

CASE 154

Stress (Takotsubo) Cardiomyopathy

1. A and C

2. A

3. C

4. B

References

Fernández-Pérez GC, Aguilar-Arjona JA, de la Fuente GT, et al: Takotsubo cardiomyopathy: assessment with cardiac MRI, *AJR Am J Roentgenol* 195(2):W139–W145, 2010.

Neil CJ, Nguyen TH, Sverdlov AL, et al: Can we make sense of takotsubo cardiomyopathy? An update on pathogenesis, diagnosis and natural history, *Expert Rev Cardiovasc Ther* 10(2):215–221, 2012.

Cross-Reference

Cardiac Imaging: The REQUISITES, ed 3, pp 294–295.

Comment

Etiology and Clinical Features

Takotsubo cardiomyopathy, or stress cardiomyopathy (other synonyms include apical ballooning syndrome and broken-heart syndrome), is a reversible cardiac dysfunction brought on by extreme stress. Takotsubo cardiomyopathy typically affects postmenopausal women. Precipitating events include the death of a loved one, financial loss, or a breakup. Patients generally have new electrocardiogram changes (e.g., ST segment elevation or T wave inversion) and elevated cardiac enzyme biomarkers that mimic myocardial infarction. Symptoms also may overlap with symptoms of myocarditis. Treatment of Takotsubo cardiomyopathy is supportive; most patients fully recover left ventricular function within months of the initial presentation.

Imaging

Echocardiography, catheter-based ventriculography, and MRI can demonstrate dyskinesis or akinesis in the mid and apical left ventricle that spares the basal segments. The heart can take on an appearance similar to a takotsubo, a bulbous Japanese pot used to catch octopi. T2-weighted MRI can show increased signal intensity, consistent with edema, which does not correspond to a vascular distribution. In contrast to acute myocardial infarction, the hyperintense T2 signal and left ventricular contraction abnormality return to normal within a few weeks after the initial presentation (Figs. A and B). Late gadolinium enhancement images typically show no myocardial enhancement (Fig. C). To make the diagnosis, obstructive coronary artery disease, myocarditis, and pheochromocytoma should be excluded.

Notes

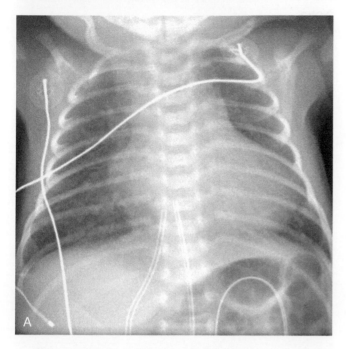

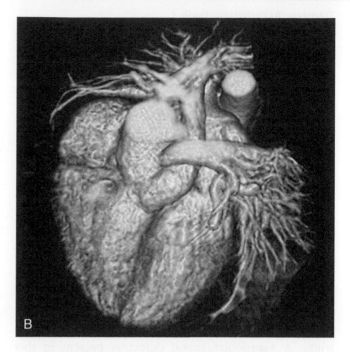

History: A 6-day-old infant presents with cyanosis and respiratory distress.

1. What should be included in the differential diagnosis? (Choose all that apply.)
   A. Transposition of the great arteries
   B. Tetralogy of Fallot
   C. Truncus arteriosus
   D. Ventricular septal defect

2. Based on the radiograph, what is the most likely diagnosis?
   A. Transposition of the great arteries
   B. Tetralogy of Fallot
   C. Truncus arteriosus
   D. Ventricular septal defect

3. What is the most common right aortic arch branching associated with this anomaly?
   A. Mirror imaging
   B. Aberrant innominate (brachiocephalic) artery
   C. Aberrant left subclavian artery
   D. Isolated left subclavian artery

4. Which of the following CT techniques would reduce radiation dose?
   A. Retrospective gating
   B. Increased z-axis
   C. Decreased tube voltage
   D. Decreased pitch

CASE 155

Truncus Arteriosus, Type I

1. A and C

2. C

3. A

4. C

Reference

Johnson TR: Conotruncal cardiac defects: a clinical imaging perspective, *Pediatr Cardiol* 31:430-437, 2010.

Cross-Reference

Cardiac Imaging: The REQUISITES, ed 3, pp 324-327.

Comment

Anatomy and Clinical Features

Truncus arteriosus is a cyanotic admixture lesion in which the pulmonary artery, aorta, and coronary arteries arise from a common trunk. There may be a main pulmonary artery, but in some patients the right and left pulmonary arteries arise separately from the common trunk. A ventricular septal defect is present in this anomaly. The truncal valve usually is tricuspid, but it can have four or more leaflets. Approximately 30% to 35% of patients have a right aortic arch, which most commonly has mirror-image branching. Truncus arteriosus is classified into different types according to the pulmonary artery anatomy. Treatment is surgical correction within the first year of life.

Associations

There is an association with DiGeorge syndrome and interrupted aortic arch. Other abnormalities may involve the coronary arteries, mitral valve, and pulmonary venous connections.

Imaging

Radiographs typically show shunt vascularity, cardiomegaly, and frequently a right-sided aortic arch (Fig. A). Echocardiography is generally adequate for diagnosis and preoperative planning in most patients. CT (Fig. B) or MRI may be performed in difficult cases to delineate the anatomy of the branch pulmonary arteries or aorticopulmonary collaterals and in patients with complex aortic arch anomalies.

Role of Imaging after Corrective Surgery

The major role of CT and MRI in truncus arteriosus is in detecting complications after corrective surgery. Important complications include right or left ventricular dysfunction, pulmonary homograft stenosis, pulmonic insufficiency, branch pulmonary artery stenosis, and neoaortic valve dysfunction.

Notes

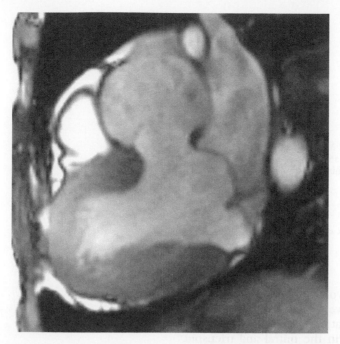

History: A 30-year-old man presents with Marfan syndrome, dilated aortic root, and mitral regurgitation.

1. Which of the following are associated with Marfan syndrome? (Choose all that apply.)
   A. Annuloaortic ectasia
   B. Dilated cardiomyopathy
   C. Mitral valve prolapse
   D. Constrictive pericarditis

2. Which disease is not associated with mitral valve prolapse?
   A. Marfan syndrome
   B. Ehlers-Danlos syndrome
   C. Polycystic kidney disease
   D. Hypertrophic cardiomyopathy

3. What is the most common cause of chordae tendineae cordis rupture in this clinical setting?
   A. Rheumatic heart disease
   B. Elongation of the chordae tendineae
   C. Iatrogenic
   D. Myocardial infarction

4. Which MRI sequence is most useful for evaluation of mitral valve prolapse?
   A. Double inversion recovery (black blood)
   B. Steady-state free precession (SSFP)
   C. Contrast-enhanced magnetic resonance angiography (MRA)
   D. Late gadolinium enhancement

Mitral Valve Prolapse

1. A and C

2. D

3. B

4. B

References

Bonow RO, Cheitlin MD, Crawford MH, et al: Task Force 3: valvular heart disease, *J Am Coll Cardiol* 45(8):1334–1340, 2005.

Enriquez-Sarano M, Akins CW, Vahanian A: Mitral regurgitation, *Lancet* 373(9672):1382–1394, 2009.

Cross-Reference

Cardiac Imaging: The REQUISITES, ed 3, pp 192–193.

Comment

Pathology and Etiology

Mitral valve prolapse can involve all components of the mitral apparatus. Mitral valve prolapse has a 5% incidence in the general population. In Marfan syndrome, congenital prolapse occurs in the mitral and tricuspid valves because the valve leaflets are redundant. If prolapse is mild, the heart may be normal. More severe prolapse may result in severe regurgitation, subacute bacterial endocarditis, chest pain, or rarely death. Geometric distortion of the left ventricle can cause moderate mitral prolapse.

Imaging Findings

Chest radiographic findings of mitral valve prolapse are similar to findings of mitral regurgitation from other causes: enlargement of the left atrium and ventricle. Mitral valve prolapse can be identified on echocardiography. Echocardiography can be used to grade the severity of prolapse and the presence and degree of regurgitation. Although angiography is not commonly performed for diagnosis, the angiographic hallmark of mitral valve prolapse is the passage of the leaflets behind the plane of the anulus into the left atrium. CT and MRI can also be used to depict the prolapsed mitral valve leaflets. The three-chamber view is ideal for this purpose (Figure).

Notes

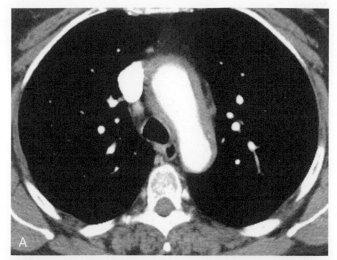

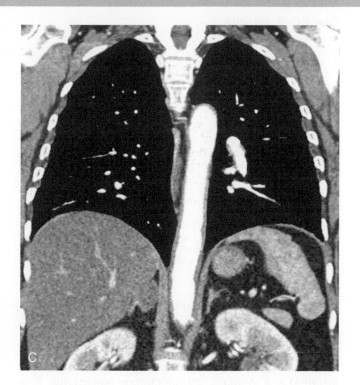

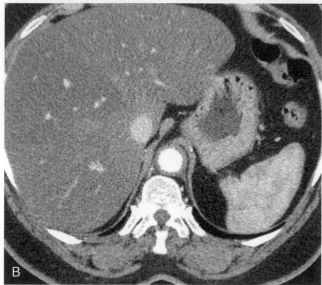

History: A 68-year-old woman presents with fatigue.

1. What should be included in the differential diagnosis? (Choose all that apply.)
   A. Giant cell arteritis
   B. Atherosclerosis
   C. Marfan syndrome
   D. Takayasu arteritis

2. Which vessel is abnormal?
   A. Aorta
   B. Renal artery
   C. Superior vena cava
   D. Inferior vena cava

3. If this patient has pain in the temples and double vision, what is the most likely diagnosis?
   A. Giant cell arteritis
   B. Atherosclerosis
   C. Marfan syndrome
   D. Takayasu arteritis

4. What is the best way to confirm the diagnosis?
   A. Temporal artery biopsy
   B. Erythrocyte sedimentation rate
   C. MRI
   D. Positron emission tomography (PET)

CASE 157

Giant Cell Arteritis

1. A and D

2. A

3. A

4. A

References

Borchers AT, Gershwin ME: Giant cell arteritis: a review of classification, pathophysiology, geoepidemiology and treatment, *Autoimmun Rev* 11(6-7):A544-A554, 2012.

Katabathina VS, Restrepo CS: Infectious and noninfectious aortitis: cross-sectional imaging findings, *Semin Ultrasound CT MR* 33(3):207-221, 2012.

Reddy GP, Gunn M, Mitsumori LM, et al: Multislice CT and MRI of the thoracic aorta. In Webb WR, Higgins CB, editors: *Thoracic imaging: pulmonary and cardiovascular radiology*, ed 2, Philadelphia, 2010, Lippincott Williams & Wilkins.

Cross-Reference

Cardiac Imaging: The REQUISITES, ed 3, p 398.

Comment

Clinical Features

Giant cell arteritis (synonyms include temporal or cranial arteritis) is a systemic granulomatous panarteritis. It is classically associated with temporal and cranial arteries, but it involves other vessels, including the aorta, coronary arteries, and mesenteric arteries. Patients can present with systemic symptoms such as fatigue or with more specific symptoms such as temporal pain, scalp tenderness, headaches, and vision disturbance. Giant cell arteritis occurs almost exclusively in patients older than 50 and is closely associated with polymyalgia rheumatica (i.e., pain and stiffness in the muscles of the pelvis and shoulders).

Diagnosis

On physical examination, temporal arteries can be hard, and the temporal pulse can be weak. Systemic inflammatory blood markers (e.g., erythrocyte sedimentation rate and C-reactive protein) are generally elevated. Temporal artery biopsy establishes the diagnosis. Prompt administration of high-dose corticosteroids is the treatment of choice because this disease is associated with sudden-onset blindness.

Imaging

MRI and CT can show dilation or stenosis of the arteries and wall thickening (Figs. A-C). MRI can show enhancement of the arterial wall or high T2 signal indicating edema. Aortic involvement is seen in about 15% of all cases of giant cell arteritis. Aortic complications seen with giant cell arteritis include aortic dissection, aortic regurgitation, and abdominal or thoracic aortic aneurysms. FDG-PET is sensitive in diagnosing active inflammation in extracranial arteries. Clinical features and patient age help differentiate giant cell arteritis from Takayasu arteritis.

Notes